COMPLICATIONS OF
FRACTURES AND
DISLOCATIONS

To Marise and my children

COMPLICATIONS OF FRACTURES AND DISLOCATIONS

Phillip M. Segelov

*Consultant Emeritus and Former Head of the
Orthopaedic Department, Liverpool Hospital and
Senior Consultant Orthopaedic Surgeon,
Fairfield Hospital, Sydney, Australia*

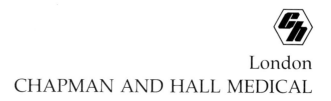

London
CHAPMAN AND HALL MEDICAL

First published in 1990 by
Chapman and Hall
11 New Fetter Lane, London EC4P 4EE

P O 1 7 3 8

Typeset in 10/12 pt Palatino by
Best-set Typesetter Ltd, Hong Kong
Printed in Great Britain at the
University Press, Cambridge

ISBN 0 412 34810 1

British Library Cataloguing in Publication Data

Segelov, Phillip M.
    Complications of fractures and dislocations.
    1. Man. Bones. Fractures. Complications
    I. Title
    617'.15

    ISBN 0-412-34810-1

Contents

Preface

The purpose of this book is to detail the common complications of fractures and dislocations, and to give an outline of their treatment. In a perfect world, the normal treatment of fractures should not allow complications to occur. However, our world is far from perfect and our treatment of fractures often falls short of the optimum. Not only this but as Robert Jones said, "Bones are not filled with marrow but with black ingratitude".

Some complications are inevitable, many are avoidable, and most can be improved with treatment. This book should help you avoid them where possible, recognize them when inevitable and treat them where practicable.

I must express my deepest appreciation to Eric Caspary, my partner and friend, for the many hours he has spent reading and correcting this book. His advice was invaluable. My thanks also to John Cumming for his fine work in illustrating the text and to the many Orthopaedic Surgeons who located radiographs used in this book. Radiographs and drawings are shown in the usual viewing position rather than in the anatomical position.

Foreword

Phillip Segelov has drawn further on his vast range of practical orthopaedic experience to write his second book, *Complications of Fractures and Dislocations*.

Complications of fracture management may be inevitable, another surgeon's, or well and truly our own problem. As one of Australia's foremost orthopaedic surgeons, and the person who first introduced advanced methods of internal fixation into Australia, no one is more qualified to explain how to avoid pitfalls, or climb out of them.

In this book, the author has achieved a lifetime's ambition. It has always been his opinion that not only are there preferred methods of treatment, but that each method has crucial turning points. For example, an operation may have many steps, but the experienced surgeon will be aware that there are only a few critical points where technique will mean the difference between success and failure.

In all parts of this book the author's selected management is indicated without hesitation or apology. Each method of treatment is fully illustrated with photographs and explanatory line drawings. Treatment regimens are covered point by point. The unique feature is the addition of text boxes of 'tips'; summaries of those essential features of the management which can make the difference between success and failure.

This book should appeal to all those who manage complications of fractures and dislocations. Trainees and younger surgeons will find the information invaluable. Experienced surgeons are likely also to find some useful surprises.

In this latest book, his love of, and skill in, surgical techniques comes to light. *If it is possible to transfer surgical experience, this book will do it.*

Eric Caspary MB,BS,FRACS
Head of Orthopaedic Department
Fairfield Hospital, Sydney

CHAPTER ONE

Introduction and general complications

1.1 INTRODUCTION

1.1.1 DEFINITION

A complication is by definition, an unexpected and unwanted change in the normal course of treatment or an unfortunate end result.

When applied to fractures and dislocations some complications are general and can occur at almost all sites whereas others are specific for that fracture or that type of treatment.

We must always bear in mind the result to be expected. In the child with the dislocated elbow shown in Fig. 1.1 we can expect full function, but half of the adults who suffer the same injury will have some permanent loss of movement and function.

Good results; some of the factors that help are

1. Age of the patient, the younger they are the more rapid and complete the recovery
2. Undisplaced fractures
3. Fractures without joint involvement
4. Dislocations without associated fractures.

Working against a good result are:

1. The age of the patient, the older the patient the more stiffness and loss of function;
2. Compound and/or comminuted and/or displaced fractures have greater soft tissue damage;
3. Joint involvement, particularly with displacement of the fragments leads to stiffness and possibly traumatic arthritis;
4. Dislocations with fractures.

1.1.2 IATROGENIC FACTORS THAT LEAD TO COMPLICATIONS

1. Poor reduction of displaced fragments (Figs 1.2 (a) and (b)) leading to malunion
2. Wrong immobilization
   (a) Plaster too short, fracture may displace (Fig. 1.3) or not unite, delayed union, non union
   (b) Plaster too long (Fig. 1.4), extra joints stiffen. Not enough padding, vascular problems, pressure sores (Fig. 1.5)
   (c) Excessive time in plaster, stiffness
   (d) Insufficient time in plaster, refracture
   (e) Poor internal fixation
   (f) Wrong choice of method (Fig. 1.6)
   (g) Poor technique (Fig. 1.7)

Remember that a radiograph that fails to reveal any fracture does not mean the limb or

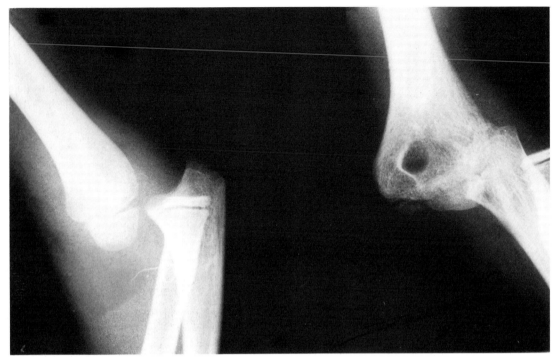

Fig. 1.1 A dislocated elbow in a child.

joint is uninjured. Soft tissue injuries such as severe ligamentous damage or rupture can have a normal radiograph. The knee joint frequently suffers damage to medial, lateral and cruciate ligaments and this can be easily overlooked.

Major complications will be discussed under the fracture in which it occurs most commonly with appropriate cross references in other fractures.

1.1.3 PLASTER IMMOBILIZATION

Plaster or its modern equivalent, the water-proof plastic casts, can in itself cause problems. Most of the problems are of our own making. The cast can be:

1. Too tight causing vascular problems (see forearm fractures; Section 2.2)

2. Too loose after the swelling goes down, allowing the fracture to displace (Fig. 1.8)
3. Poorly applied so that pressure sores can occur where the plaster presses and rubs

Key points in cast application

1. Never apply a full cast on a recent fracture. Use slabs which only encompass two thirds of the circumference or split the full cast and open it so that it acts as a supporting shell only.
2. Always use padding over the pressure points to allow for swelling.
3. If you use slabs and a crepe bandage you can tighten the slabs with elastoplast at one week or alternatively, complete the cast.
4. Always hold the limb in the final position during application of the cast. Flexing the elbow or dorsiflexing the foot after the cast

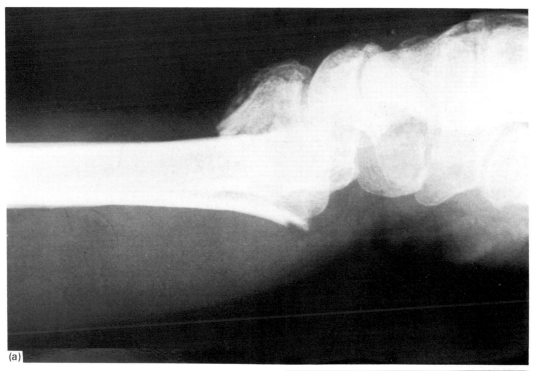

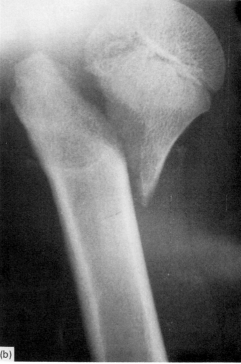

Figs 1.2 (a) Lateral radiograph of a displaced Colle's fracture of the wrist and (b) AP of a displaced fracture of the upper third of the humerus.

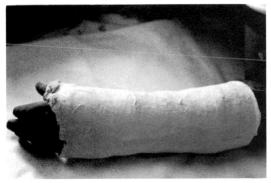

Fig. 1.3 This patient has a fracture of the shaft of the radius and ulna, the plaster should extend above the elbow to control pronation and supination.

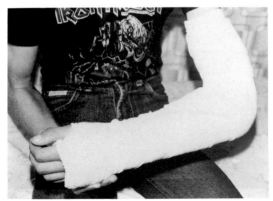

Fig. 1.4 This plaster has been applied for a Colles' fracture of the wrist and extends above the elbow unnecessarily.

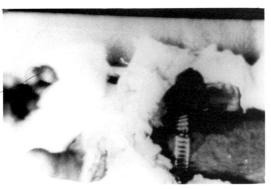

Fig. 1.5 This plaster was too tight and swelling and pain in the hand caused the plaster to be removed. Note the metallic watch band which had not been removed and was helping to compromise the circulation.

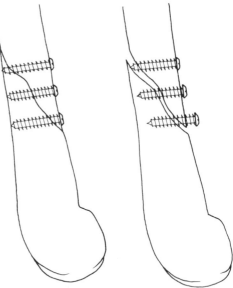

Fig. 1.6 This fracture of the humerus cannot be immobilized with three screws alone (a plate giving fixation above and below the fracture is necessary). Note how the fixation is lost and the fracture bends and often fails to unite.

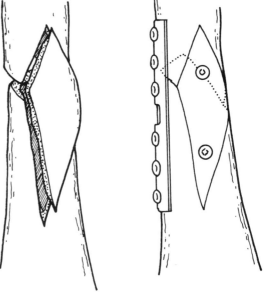

Fig. 1.7 This fracture has been well reduced and plated but the plate is far too short and the fracture will redisplace. If this happens you have lost the whole reason for operating on this patient.

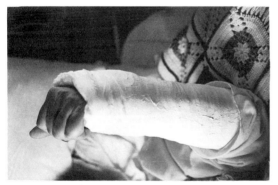

Fig. 1.8 This full short arm plaster is too loose and will allow the fracture to redisplace.

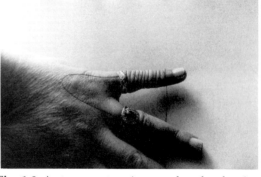

Fig. 1.9 A strong suture is passed under the ring and wound around the finger distal to the ring.

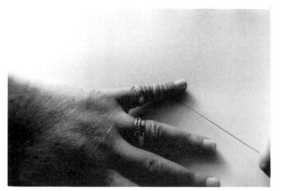

Fig. 1.10 Unwinding the thread (which can be lubricated with soap after application) from the proximal end moves the ring down the finger and over the joints.

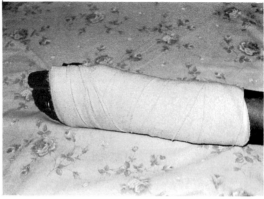

Fig. 1.11 This patient has a Colles' fracture. Dorsal and radial slabs have been applied over padding and are held on by a lightly stretched crepe bandage. Later the fixation can be tightened without removal by an elastoplast adhesive bandage.

material is applied creates a ridge which can block the circulation or cause a pressure sore.
5. Make sure your assistant does not leave finger or thumb prints in the cast.

1.2 GENERAL COMPLICATIONS

1.2.1 SOME COMMON COMPLICATIONS

(i) Post-reduction swelling

All fractures are associated with swelling at and distal to the fracture site and allowance must be made for this in applying immobi-

lization. The following rules will help you avoid problems.

1. Always remove rings, bangles and watches on the injured limb. Rings if tight can often be removed after anaesthesia or analgesia by the thread method (Figs 1.9 and 1.10) or even with a ring cutter.
2. Always apply padding to all fractures before application of plaster. There is no place for unpadded plasters in the management of fractures.
3. No recent fracture should be immobilized in a full plaster. In the upper limb single or double slabs should be used (Fig. 1.11). In

lower limb fractures, a full plaster can be applied but should be immediately split along its full length.

4. All fractured limbs should be elevated for 12–24 hours. Movement of the fingers and toes must be done actively by the patient.
5. Severe pain, swelling, blueness of digits and loss of feeling are signs that the plaster is too tight. If in doubt split the plaster or bandages down to the skin, elevate and start active movement. If there is not a rapid improvement then a fasciotomy may be necessary (Chapter 2.3.1 (d) (ii) and Chapter 4.2.3 (iv)).

(ii) Swelling, pain and stiffness

Some swelling and stiffness is present in all fractures after removal of plaster in adults but is often absent in children.

All adult fractures:

1. have significant soft tissue damage around the fracture site;
2. lose muscle bulk and muscle power in plaster;
3. swell rapidly on dependency;
4. have some stiffness of joints that have been immobilized and some discomfort on movement.

'Fracture disease' is a term used to describe what can happen after fractures in the limbs. In this condition the limb (usually the leg) has chronic oedema, soft tissue atrophy, joint stiffness and osteoporosis. This occurs as a result of prolonged loss of function associated with the fracture, reaction to the fracture and the immobilization. Oedema can become fixed and invaded by fibrous tissue with resultant thickening of tissues and loss of movement and function.

To prevent these problems:

1. Immobilize the limb for the minimum time
2. Elevate the limb for periods during day and night
3. Support the limb with elastic support after plaster removal
4. Exercise the limb actively and regularly
5. Encourage protected and progressive weight bearing and return to normal function.

Often 'fracture disease' occurs in cases of fractures of the tibia and fibula that are slow to unite. This problem can be avoided by internal fixation of the fracture giving stability and allowing early return of function including weight bearing.

1.2.2 DELAYED UNION AND NON UNION

(i) Delayed union

This is defined as being a delay in the normal timing of bone union. It is an arbitrary figure and each fracture will need to be considered on its merits. However, if a fracture has taken one and a half times the normal time and is still not steadily progressing toward union then there is delay in union of the fracture.

Table 1.1 gives a rough guide to the normal range for clinical union of common fractures in children and adults.

Please note:

1. With children, the younger they are the quicker union occurs. You can halve the children's times for union as given below where the child is under one year old.
2. Clinical union precedes full radiological union by a large time margin. Clinical union is judged by stability and loss of tenderness at the fracture site. The radiograph picture should show callus and obliteration of the fracture line.

(ii) Non union

An arbitrary time limit has to be put on the process of bone union. Beyond this point it is unlikely that the fracture will unite without

TABLE 1.1 Normal range for clinical union of common fractures in children and adults.

Clinical union	Children (wks)	Adults (wks)
Phalanges	2–3	3–4
Metacarpals	2–3	3–4
Bennett's	2–3	3–4
Colles'	3	4–5
Smiths	3	4–6
Forearm	3–4	6–8
Head of radius	3	4
Olecranon	3	4–6
Supracondylar humerus	3	4–6
Shaft of humerus	4–6	8
Neck of humerus	3	5
Clavicle	3	6
Scapula	3	5–6
Pelvis-Pubic rami	3	5–6
Femur-shaft	6	14–16
Tibia	6–8	14
Ankle	6	8–12

TREATMENT

Delayed union is managed by providing better stability at the fracture site and by bone grafting. In most cases treatment will involve open reduction and internal fixation using compression techniques where possible, and bone grafting. This is discussed after Non union.

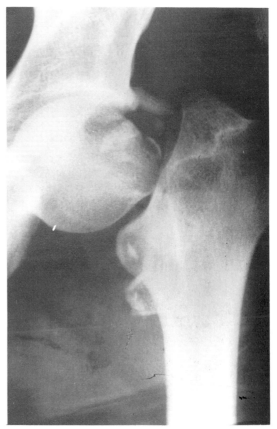

Fig. 1.12 This patient has a displaced subcapital fracture of the neck of the femur, a fracture that frequently damages the blood supply to the head of the femur.

help. The time limit is generally considered to be two to three times the normal time for union of the fracture.

There is a natural tendency for bones to unite even if fractures are only given minimal treatment, however to get the fracture to unite without shortening, or angulation often creates problems including delayed and non union.

What is needed for bone union is that:

1. Both ends of the bones at the fracture site have good blood supply.
2. There is stability at the fracture site.
3. Apposition of the bone fragments.

Fig. 1.12 is an example of a fracture that could go on to delayed or non union due to poor blood supply at the fracture site. (There is also no bony apposition and no stability.)

Fig. 1.13 shows an example of failure to unite due to lack of continued immobilization.

The radiographs do show us some differences at the fracture site. There is the hyper-

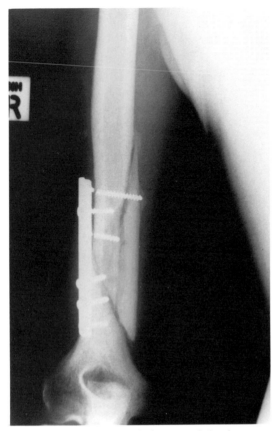

Fig. 1.13 When internal fixation fails fractures commonly go on to non union.

trophic non union (Figs 1.14(a) and (b)), where nature is desperately trying to stabilize the fracture and makes more and more callus to try and bridge the gap.

There is the much less dramatic fracture of the atrophic non union (Fig. 1.15(a) and (b)), which is usually associated with poor blood supply. The fracture site is on strike and it looks as though nothing is happening on the radiographs for month after month.

You cannot expect bone to jump a gap, so that a missing piece of bone must be bridged or non union will occur (Fig. 1.16).

Infection at a fracture site will interfere both with the stability of the fixation and the blood supply to the bone ends and may also lead to non union (Fig. 1.17).

Iatrogenic causes are not uncommon.

If we hold a fracture apart with a plate and screws then the plate will either break at the fracture site or become loose at one end and we will lose stability and our opportunity for union (Figs 1.18(a) and (b)).

If we strip the central fragment in a segmental butterfly fracture we can rob it of its blood supply and create a non union (Fig. 1.19).

If our fixation is poor, such as with a loose plaster (Fig. 1.20), or a loose nail non union may result.

Treatment of delayed union and non union union.

1. Restore stability. If you have an unstable fracture trying desperately to unite, such as a fracture with hypertrophic non union (Fig. 1.14), then you restore stability by open reduction and compression plating.

KEY POINTS

a. **Use an adequate incision, do not strip the periosteum.**
b. **There is no need to interfere with the fracture site and remove the tissue between the bone ends. This tissue will convert to bone when stability is provided (Fig. 1.21(a) and (b)).**
c. **Use a plate of adequate length on the compression side of the bone, the medial side of the tibia, the lateral side of the femur.**
d. **Start the rehabilitation of the limb immediately with support and active exercise followed in a few weeks by graduated weight bearing.**
e. **In these circumstances there is no need for a bone graft, however if in doubt use a bone graft (Fig. 1.22) (see later).**

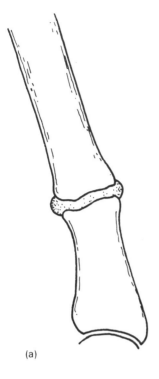

(a)

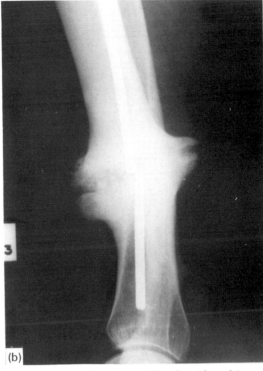

(b)

Figs 1.14 (a) and (b) Hypertrophic non union in a fracture of the tibia 'immobilized' with a thin nail which has broken. Note the exuberant callus as nature tries desperately to immobilize the fracture.

2. Bone grafting
   (a) Bone grafting using cancellous bone from the internal aspect of the iliac crest is advised in all cases of delayed union and non union where hypertropic changes are not present (Fig. 1.26).
   (b) Other indications for bone grafting include:
      (i) Filling a defect in bone (Fig. 1.23).
      (ii) Reinforcing the cortex opposite the plate in a comminuted fracture (Fig. 1.24(a)).
      (iii) Supporting a butterfly fragment (Fig. 1.24(b)).

KEY POINTS
---

a. Autologous cancellous bone grafting is the preferred form of bone grafting. Bank bone or heterologous grafting is not as good but may be used.

b. Cortical bone grafting is not advised. Cortical bone is slow to incorporate and to become revascularized. In the past cortical grafts were used for stability as well as for stimulation of bone growth. They were poor at both functions.

c. The bed into which the graft is placed should if possible be of good vascularity.

d. Petalling (Fig. 1.25), a partial decortication of cortical bone improves the vascular bed for the graft.

e. Bone grafts can be obtained

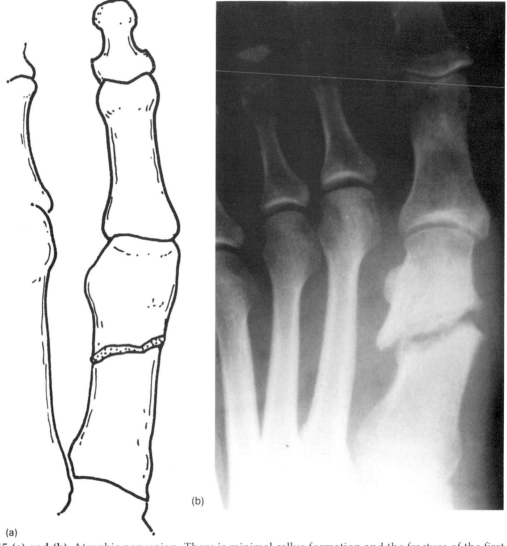

(a) (b)

Figs 1.15 (a) and (b) Atrophic non union. There is minimal callus formation and the fracture of the first metatarsal is indolent and unchanging over many months.

from a number of sites (Fig. 1.26). The common areas are the inner table of the iliac crest, the upper end of the tibia, the greater trochanter and the distal end of the radius.

Bone grafts need to be protected from the heat of the operating theatre light and should not be put in normal saline as this will kill off some of the cells. The best technique is to take the graft at a stage when the cancellous material can be taken from its original bed and placed directly into the operation site.

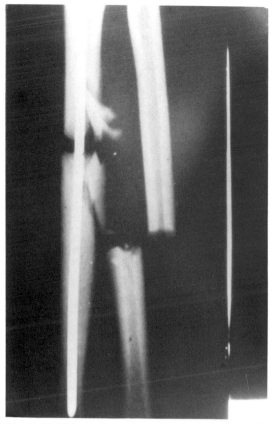

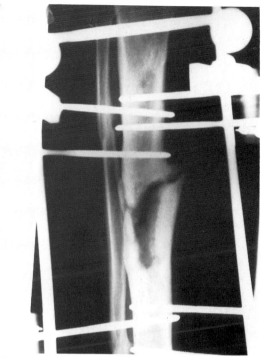

Fig. 1.17 Anteroposterior radiograph of a compound fracture of the tibia in which there is active infection. Note the external fixation and the defect in the tibia.

Fig. 1.16 This patient has the fractures of the radius and ulna held apart so that union will never occur.

Iliac crest grafts should be used when a large amount of bone is required, say in fractures of the femur (Fig. 1.27).

Cancellous grafting from the proximal end of the tibia (Fig. 1.26) should be the standard procedure where grafting is required in tibial fractures. A surprising amount of bone is available and there is the advantage of not having an extra area involved.

The greater trochanter is a not a good donor site. There have been case reports of fractures of the neck of the femur after its use. The area is so close to the iliac crest that you should use the crest for preference as this is the better site.

The distal end of the radius can be used in such procedures as grafting the carpal scaphoid. Here a small block of cancellous bone or a small quantity of cancellous chips can be harvested.

(iii) Infection and delayed union

Occasionally we see a low grade infection around a fracture usually where there has been internal fixation. The clinical picture is one of a persistent sinus draining pus that is often sterile. This picture can be associated with delayed union.

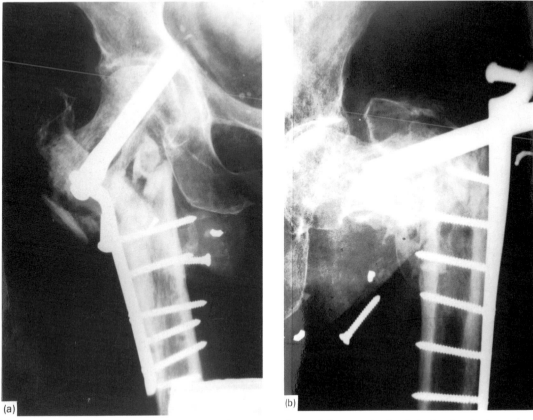

Figs 1.18 (a) and (b) Poor fixation system for a comminuted fracture in the intertrochanteric region of the femur. Failure was inevitable.

TREATMENT

1. Accept that union is going to be slow and continue immobilization, dressings and antibiotics when there is a sensitive organism cultured. Care should be taken to keep the infection under control so as to avoid a chronic osteomyelitis developing.
2. If there is internal fixation and it is stable (no loosening of screws), then leave the plate and screws in situ and await union. The delay will probably be an extra 50% in time to obtain union.
3. Cancellous grafts can be added to a fracture site even in the presence of mild infection.
4. Once the fracture has united then the plates and screws can be removed and any bone infection can be dealt with by sequestrectomy and debridement.

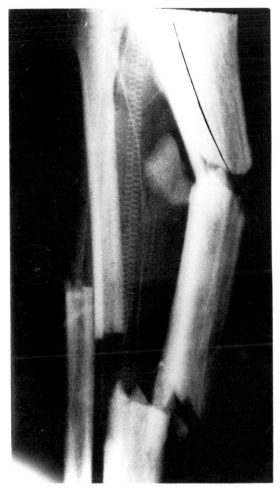

Fig. 1.19 Segmental fracture of the tibia.

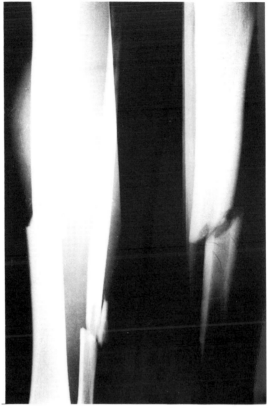

Fig. 1.20 Non union of a distal third fracture of the tibia due to poor immobilization in a loose plaster.

(iv) Infection and non union

There are particular problems with this condition. Quite often as a consequence of the infection the screws loosen and stability is lost at the fracture site. The plate acts as a loose foreign body. Infection will not clear up and the fracture will not unite whilst there is instability and a foreign body.

TREATMENT _____

1. **Remove all loose internal fixation**
2. **Remove all dead bone**
3. **Remove all necrotic soft tissue and if the infection is severe set up a suction and irrigation system**
4. **Stabilize the fracture with external fixation if possible (Fig. 1.28). If**

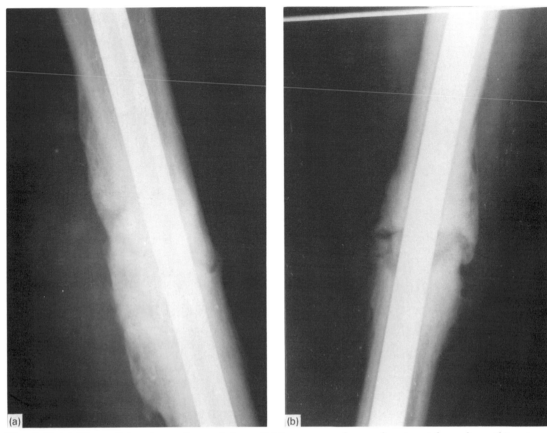

Figs 1.21 (a) The nail has been changed for a thicker one and sound union takes place; (b) antero-posterior radiographs of an ununited fracture of the femur with a loose medullary nail.

this is not possible then apply a plaster and consider stabilizing the fracture internally when the wound has healed

5. **When the wounds have healed or have improved to the point where there is a healthy bed for a graft, consider decortication of the bone ends and the insertion of a cancellous bone graft (Fig. 1.29)**

1.2.3 PATHOLOGICAL FRACTURES

A pathological fracture is a fracture through an area of abnormal bone. The bony abnormality can be biochemical such as in rickets, metabolic such as in postmenopausal osteoporosis or the lipidoses, or (more commonly) due to a benign cyst or tumour (Fig. 1.30), or primary or secondary malignant lesion (Fig. 1.31). Another rare cause of pathological fractures is osteomyelitis.

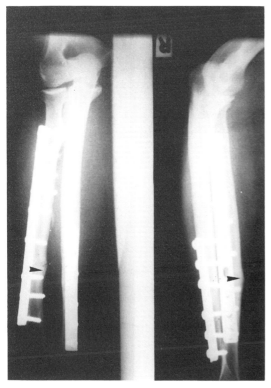

Fig. 1.22 In forearm fractures requiring plating it is always advisable to use a bone graft.

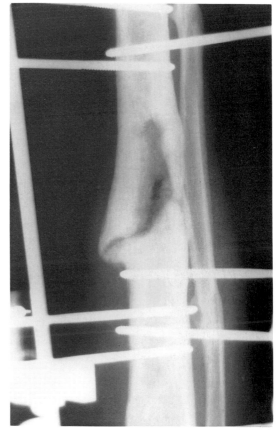

Fig. 1.23 When all the infection has cleared this defect in the tibia required bone grafting.

Fractures associated with malignant tumours are not uncommon and have particular problems as the patient's life span can be very limited, with pain and loss of mobility. Malignant pathological fractures will not unite unless there is some adjuvant treatment of the malignant process (Fig. 1.32).

TREATMENT

1. **Establish the cause of the pathological process by means of radiograph, bone scan, CT scan. Very often open or needle biopsy may be necessary to establish the nature of the lesion.**
2. **Benign lesions will heal often with the help of a bone graft to fill a defect (Fig. 1.33).**
3. **Remember the most common tumours to metastasize to bone are from primary tumours in lung, prostate, breast, kidney and**

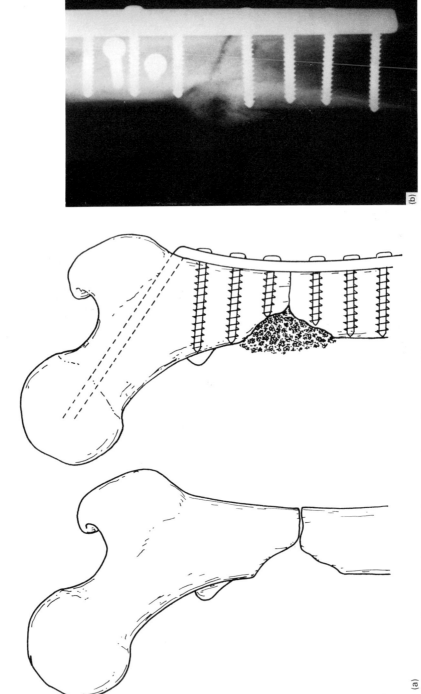

Fig. 1.24 (a) Always reinforce a defect opposite a plate caused by comminution or a missing fragment otherwise the plate will break; (b) bone grafting a butterfly segment of a femur.

(a)

(b)

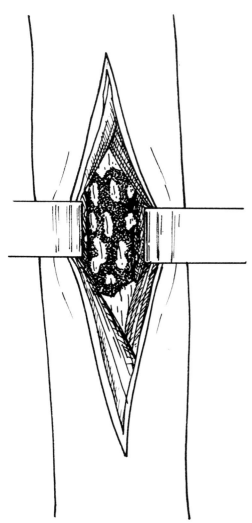

Fig. 1.25 Petalling or decortication of the shaft of a long bone.

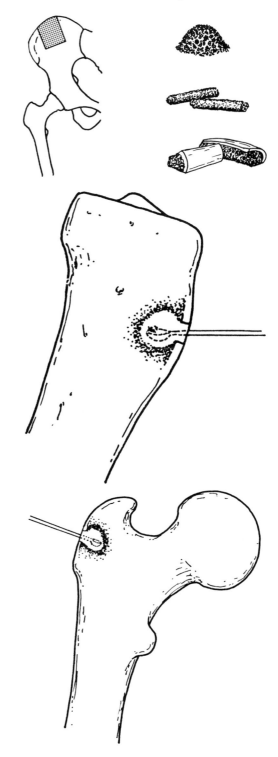

Fig. 1.26 The sites commonly used for obtaining cancellous bone for bone grafting.

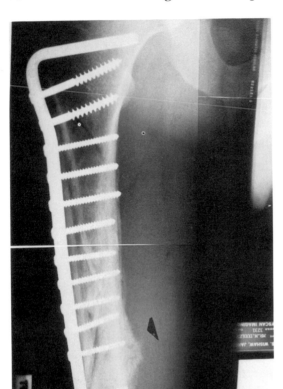

Fig. 1.27 Comminuted fracture of the femur supported on the medial side by a cancellous graft after plating.

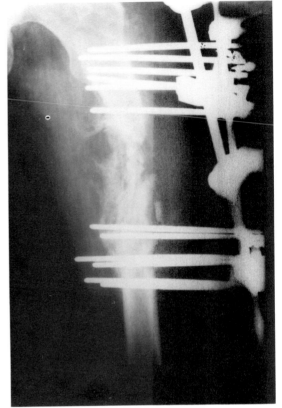

Fig. 1.29 Anteroposterior radiograph of an infected fracture of the femur after removal of sequestra and subsequent grafting. Note the external fixateur.

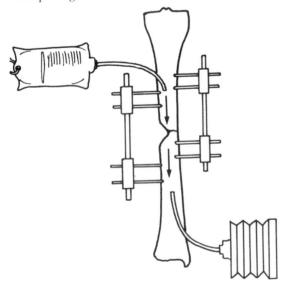

Fig. 1.28 Compound fracture of the tibia with external fixation after debridement and with a suction irrigation system in place.

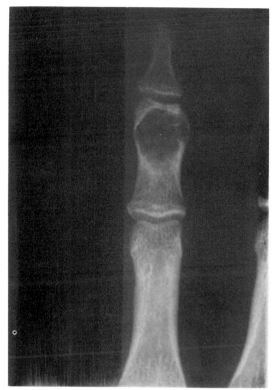

Fig. 1.30 This cystic lesion in the middle phalanx of the little finger has thinned the cortex so that very minor trauma will cause a fracture. An enchondroma.

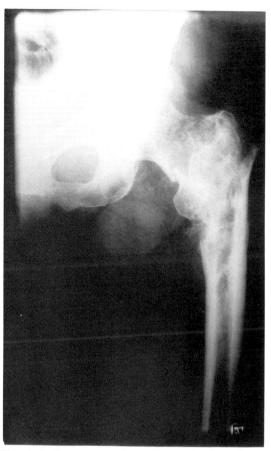

Fig. 1.31 Anteroposterior radiograph of a subtrochanteric fracture of the femur in a patient who has bilateral subtrochanteric fractures due to metastases from carcinoma of the breast.

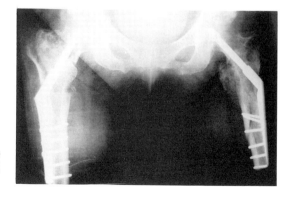

Fig. 1.32 The same patient as in Fig. 1.31. The fractures are uniting after treatment and internal fixation.

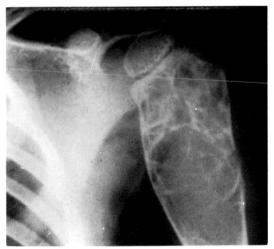

Fig. 1.33 This huge simple cyst of the humerus has been filled with a cancellous bone graft to assist it to consolidate.

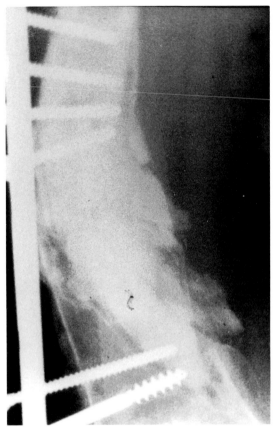

Fig. 1.34 Bone cement has been used to fill a defect but the fixation has failed.

thyroid. **Examine these areas clinically and on radiograph and with other appropriate tests.**

4. **Fractures associated with secondary malignant lesions generally will not heal. If possible they should be treated aggressively by internal fixation with long plates or rods to bypass the structural defect.**

   Bone cement or ceramic spacers can be used to fill in defects and improve bone strength so that the patient can be mobilized (**Fig. 1.34**). There is a strong case for prophylactically inserting intramedullary rods in femoral metastases (**Fig. 1.35**).

5. **The primary tumour may require treatment, and radiotherapy may be important in controlling the local disease and allowing bone union to proceed.**

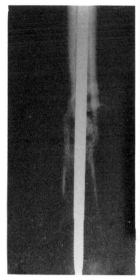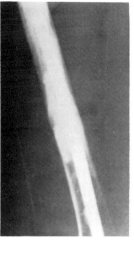

Fig. 1.35 Medullary nail has been inserted prophylactically in this femur which has metastases from a carcinoma of the breast.

1.2.4 REFRACTURES

Refracture of a bone is uncommon. Of all fractures less than 2% break again at the same point. When it does occur the patient (or the parents) are concerned that there is a lack of calcium in the bones making the bones brittle. This is usually not the case. The refracture is due to:

1. Insufficient immobilization to allow union.
2. Failure to allow the bone to return to full strength before stressing it. We remove the cast or cease immobilization before full union occurs to allow early return of movement and to strengthen the muscles and ultimately the bone. This does not mean that the bone is ready to be tested by running, jumping, falling etc.
3. An injury similar to the original one that caused the first fracture.

TREATMENT

It is unusual for a refracture at the same site of injury to displace significantly. Immobilization in a cast for an equivalent period as was used in the first fracture plus one or two weeks is all that is necessary.

Displaced fractures are treated on their merits as an individual fracture.

Refracture after open reduction, plating and subsequent removal of the plate is usually due to:

1. **Removing the plate too soon. Allow at least one year for the bone to consolidate and for the line of weight bearing and stress to bypass the plate (Fig. 1.36).**
2. **After removal of a plate allow six to eight weeks of restricted activity to give the screw holes time to fill in. Avoid body contact sports for ten to twelve weeks. If refracture does occur replating may be necessary in lower limb fractures.**

1.2.5 MULTIPLE FRACTURES AND BRITTLE BONES

Osteogenesis imperfecta does exist both in the florid form (Fig. 1.37), and more subtly in a child with blue sclera and bones that break more easily.

The gross disease will require expert treatment with rodding of the long bones (Fig. 1.38). The more subtle variety will have a varying number of fractures in early childhood which will require treatment on the merits of each fracture. Fortunately in the milder form of the disease the tendency of the bones to fracture lessens as they reach maturity. Often they reach adult life with a history of ten to twenty different fractures and are then free of further troubles.

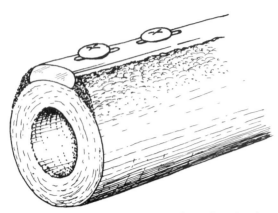

Fig. 1.36 Section of a bone with a plate in situ. Note that the plate has been bypassed by a ridge of bone on each side. This is a sign that the plate can safely be removed.

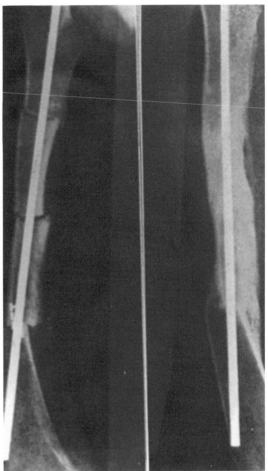

Fig. 1.38 Rodding the femur after multiple corrective osteotomies.

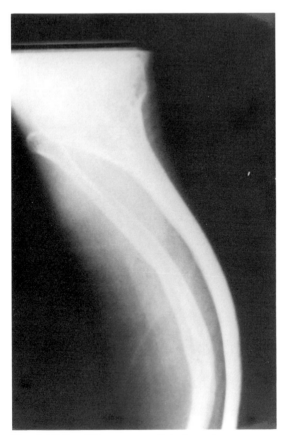

Fig. 1.37 Fragilitas osseum thin bone type.

FURTHER READING

Non union

Weber, B. G. and Cech, O. (1976) *Pseudarthrosis.* Hans Huber, Bern.

Muller, M. E., Allgower, M., Schneider, R. and Willinegger, H. (1979) *Manual of Internal Fixation.* 2nd edn, Springer-Verlag, New York.

Pathological fractures

Rockwood, C. A. and Green, D. P. (1984) *Fractures in Adults.* 2nd edn, J.B. Lippincott, Philadelphia.

Haberman, E. T. (1980) Review of 125 Cases of Pathological Fractures, *Orthop. Tran.*, **4**, 346–354.

Osteogenesis imperfecta

Bauze, R. J., Smith, R. and Francis, M. J. O. (1975) A new look at osteogenesis imperfecta. A clinical, radiological and biochemical study of forty two patients, *J. Bone Joint Surg.* (Br), **57-B**, 2–12.

CHAPTER TWO

Fractures of the upper limb

2.1 FINGERS, METACARPALS AND WRIST

2.1.1 FINGERS

(a) Distal phalanx

(i) Non union

Comminuted fractures of the distal phalanges with separation (the injury that occurs with crushing) often unite only with fibrous union. This is of no importance as firm fibrous union will still allow full function. Local tenderness often persists for several months (Fig. 2.1).

(ii) Nail bed injuries

A large percentage of fractures are compound through the nail bed and there is often damage to the nail bed. Permanent nail deformities may result. These injuries should be cleaned and repaired under magnification so that accurate repair of the nail bed occurs minimizing any scarring of the nail. Use the nail as a splint.

Where deformity is gross, ablation of the nail bed may be necessary (Fig. 2.2).

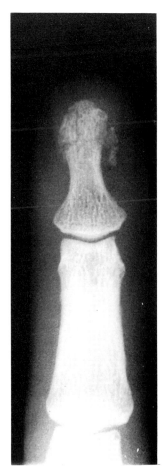

Fig. 2.1 Anteroposterior radiograph of a comminuted fracture of the distal phalanx of an index finger. The separated fragments may not unite by bony union.

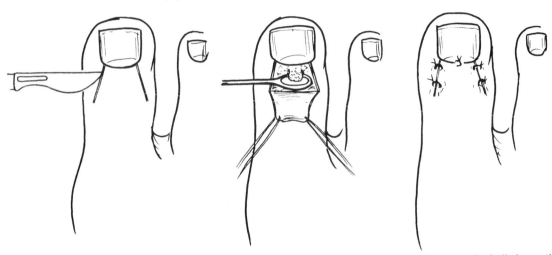

Fig. 2.2 The steps in ablation of the nail bed. Note the incision and the careful removal of all the nail matrix including the corners.

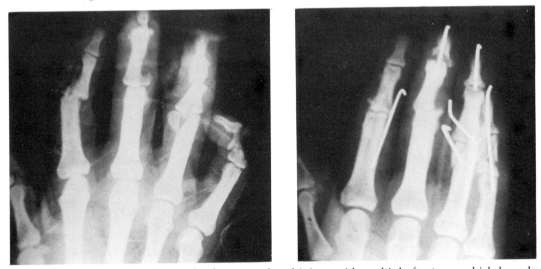

Fig. 2.3 Anteroposterior radiograph of a severe hand injury with multiple fractures which have been held in place with K-wires. Defects have been filled with bone grafts.

KEY POINTS

a. **Raise a flap with a wide base proximally.**
b. **Make a central cut through the nail bed to the bone.**
c. **Carefully dissect the two halves of the nail bed from the bone.**
d. **Curette out the nail folds.**

(b) Proximal and middle phalanges

(i) Non union

Phalangeal fractures usually unite in four weeks and only present a problem if there is missing bone. In these cases a bone graft and stabilizing wires or small screws may be necessary (Fig. 2.3).

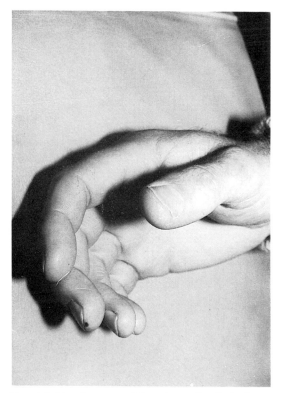

Fig. 2.4 Hand at rest. Note how the little finger rotates towards the base of the thumb.

(ii) Malunion

This is a much more common and serious problem as the hand will only work as a functional unit if the axial and rotary alignment is correct. Remember that as the fingers flex the middle, ring and little fingers progressively rotate so that they point towards the base of the thumb (Fig. 2.4).

TREATMENT

Where a fracture has united with rotary deformity giving 'blocking' of the normal flexion action of the fingers, a corrective osteotomy should be done (Fig. 2.5).

> ### KEY POINTS
> a. **Use a dorsal incision on the ulnar side of the finger except for the little finger where the incision is dorsal and radial.**
> b. **It is always easier to correct deformity where it occurs, namely the fracture site.**
> c. **Stabilize the correction with Kirschner wires or other internal fixation.**

(c) Finger fractures with instability

Many sporting injuries cause severe damage to the base of a phalanx and create interphalangeal joint instability (Fig. 2.6). The primary treatment of such fractures should, where possible, stabilize the joint.

TREATMENT

Permanent instability and traumatic arthritis may be indications for either fusion of the joint (Fig. 2.7) or more rarely joint replacement.

2.1.2 METACARPALS

Fractures of the neck of the metacarpals commonly have a flexion deformity and unite in this position (Fig. 2.8). Attempts at reduction often fail as there is comminution and impaction of the cortex on the flexor aspect and nothing to support the head of the metacarpal in the reduced postion (Fig. 2.9).

This residual deformity is of little consequence as there is such a large articular surface that there is no loss of function, only loss of prominence of the knuckle.

Fractures of the shaft of the metacarpals are unstable if multiple and can lead to malunion.

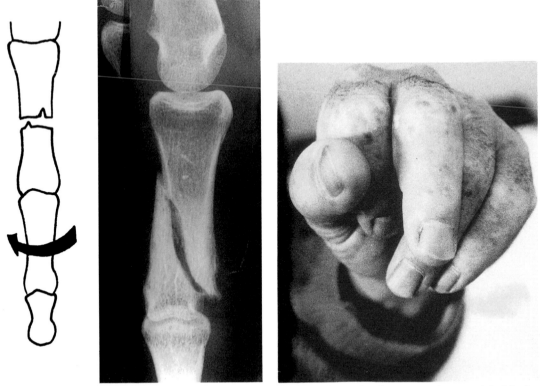

Fig. 2.5 Malrotated fracture of the proximal phalanx. Note how the finger overlaps and is blocked during flexion.

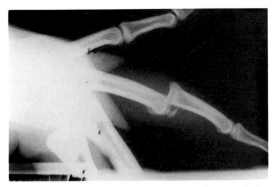

Fig. 2.6 Fracture dislocation of the base of the proximal phalanx showing the joint damage.

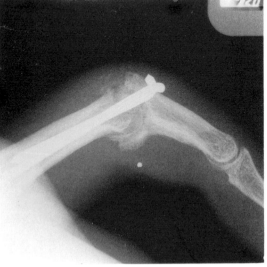

Fig. 2.7 Lateral radiograph of the proximal interphalangeal (PIP) joint which is undergoing arthrodesis after severe damage in a fracture dislocation.

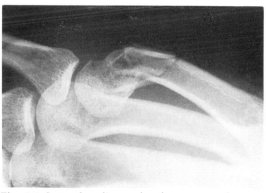

Fig. 2.8 Lateral radiograph of a commonly seen fracture of the neck of the fifth metacarpal with flexion deformity.

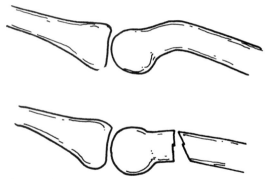

Fig. 2.9 Sketch showing how the neck of the metacarpal is unsupported after reduction.

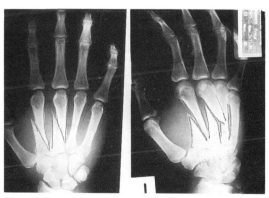

Fig. 2.10 Malunited fractures of metacarpal shafts. After osteotomy the correction can be held by a small external fixateur.

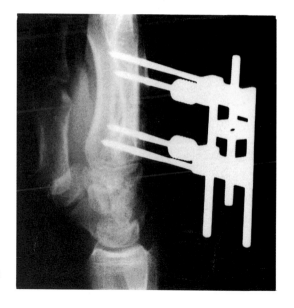

TREATMENT OF MALUNION

Osteotomy of the metacarpals at the fracture site with internal or external fixation (Kirschner wires) to maintain the position (Fig. 2.10).

Fractures of the base of the metacarpals are unstable if multiple or if it is the base of the fifth metacarpal. There is often dorsal displacement which if it persists causes the whole finger ray to point in a volar direction upsetting the plane of the metacarpal heads.

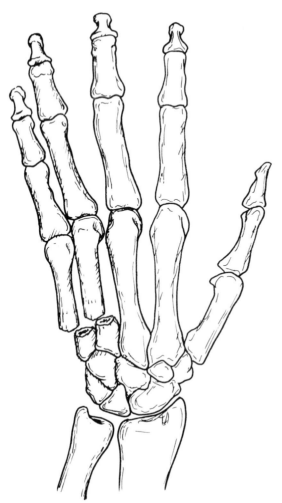

Fig. 2.11 Fractures or fracture dislocations of the base of the metacarpals cause alignment problems and must be reduced and pinned.

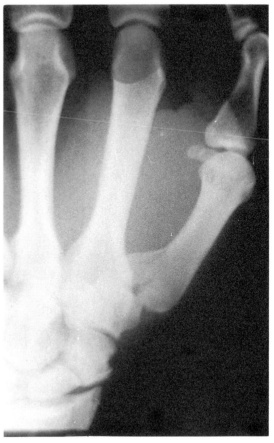

Fig. 2.12 Anteroposterior radiograph of a Bennett's fracture with some displacement.

TREATMENT

The deformity must be corrected by an osteotomy at the fracture site with appropriate fixation with Kirschner wires (Fig. 2.11).

(a) Bennett's fracture

Bennett's fracture is a fracture of the base of the first metacarpal involving the carpometa-carpal joint. There is commonly subluxation of this joint. There can be:

(i) Malunion

This fracture often unites with a degree of malunion but with little functional impairment (Fig. 2.12). Angulation of the fracture whilst not ideal can be accepted.

(ii) Persistent subluxation

This is much more important and is believed to be a major factor in the development of a traumatic arthritis in manual workers.

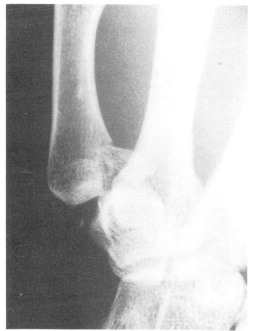

Fig. 2.13 Bennett's fracture with subluxation, poor position.

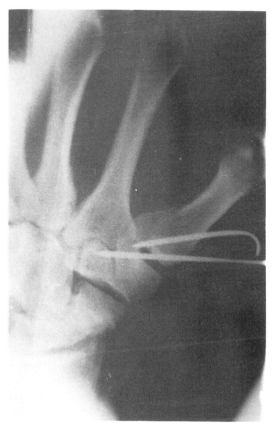

Fig. 2.14 Percutaneous pins hold the fracture seen in Fig. 2.13 in perfect position.

TREATMENT

The best treatment is prevention. Do not accept poor reduction (Fig. 2.13). Closed percutaneous pinning is the treatment of choice (Fig. 2.14).

(iii) Traumatic arthritis

This condition usually comes on many years after the original fracture. Arthritis of this joint is by no means confined to those who have had fractures.

The clinical picture is that of a middle aged to elderly person (usually male) with some prominence of the base of the first metacarpal and localized pain in this area. Often grating can be palpated when the thumb is moved. Radiographs will confirm the deformity of the base of the proximal phalanx and the degeneration of the joint (Fig. 2.15).

TREATMENT

Once the symptoms warrant operative treatment there are three possibilities.

1. Excision arthroplasty. This is a good pain relieving operation but does give some weakness of the thumb. It should be used in the older person or in sedentary workers.

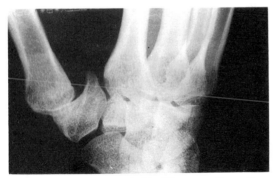

Fig. 2.15 Traumatic arthritis 20 years after a Bennett's fracture.

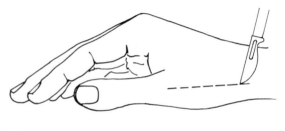

(a)

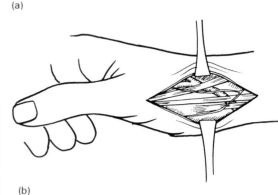

(b)

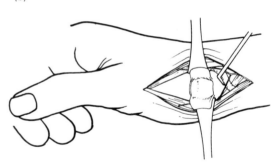

(c)

Fig. 2.16 (a) the skin incision for operations on the trapezium; (b) the position of the dorsal branch the radial nerve; (c) the capsular incision and shelling out the trapezium. Note the proximity of the radial artery.

KEY POINTS

a. to preserve the dorsal branch of the radial nerve after making a 5 cm radial incision (Fig. 2.16 (a) and (b))
b. as you go deeper to preserve the radial artery (Fig. 2.16(c)).
c. to carefully shell out the trapezium preserving the flexor carpi radialis tendon which is closely applied to the deep aspect of the trapezium (Fig. 2.16(c)).
d. fill the space left with local soft tissue or a piece of extensor carpi radialis tendon (Fig. 2.17).

TREATMENT

2. **Arthrodesis of the carpometacarpal joint is an excellent pain relieving operation which maintains the strength of the thumb at the expense of some mobility. The operation needs careful attention.**

KEY POINTS

a. to preserve the dorsal branch of the radial nerve after making 5 cm radial incision (Fig. 2.16 (a) and (b)).

b. as you go deeper to preserve the radial artery (Fig. 2.16(c)).
c. excise the joint surfaces and apply a small T-plate.
d. splay the screws in the T-plate to get better fixation (Fig. 2.18).

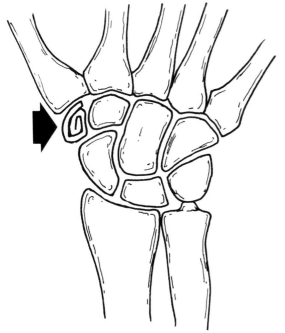

Fig. 2.17 Soft tissue interposition after excision of the trapezium. Note the piece of tendon coiled in the space.

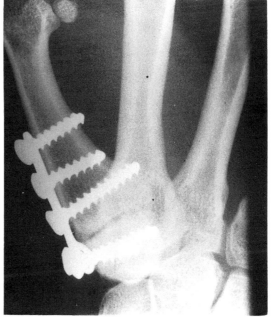

Fig. 2.18 Arthrodesis of the joint between the trapezium and the first metacarpal.

TREATMENT

3. **Replacement arthroplasty theoretically gives the best of both worlds in that there is stability as well as loss of pain. However the operation is by no means always successful and dislocation of the prosthesis must be prevented by careful capsular repair and reinforcement.**

┌─── **KEY POINTS** ───────────┐

a. to preserve the dorsal branch of the radial nerve after making a 5 cm radial incision (Fig. 2.16(a) and (b)).

b. as you go deeper to preserve the radial artery (Fig. 2.16(c)).

c. carefully shell out the trapezium preserving the flexor carpi radialis tendon on the deep aspect.

d. drill the hole in the base of the first metacarpal to seat the prosthesis.

e. reconstruct the capsule thoroughly and reinforce it with a slip of the flexor carpi radialis tendon (Fig. 2.19).

└──────────────────────────────┘

Which operation should be done in any one patient? This depends on the age and the

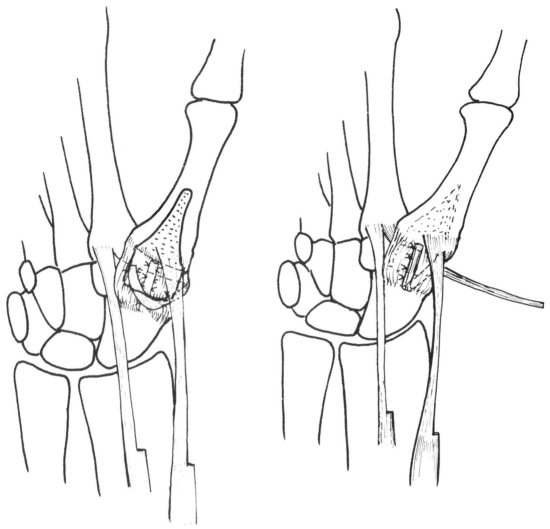

Fig. 2.19 This diagram shows prosthetic replacement of the trapezium. Note the reinforcement of the capsule.

activity level. A general guide would be as follows:

1. Excision arthroplasty, for sedentary workers and retired people.
2. Arthrodesis for young manually active people.
3. Arthroplasty for middle aged moderately active people.

2.1.3 WRIST

(a) Colles' fracture in adults

(i) Malunion

This is probably the most frequent complication in one of the most common fractures that we see. There are three types of malunion:

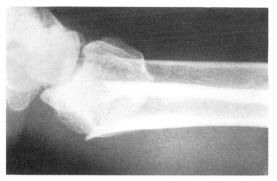

Fig. 2.20 Lateral radiograph of a malunited Colles' fracture. Note the dorsal angulation and displacement.

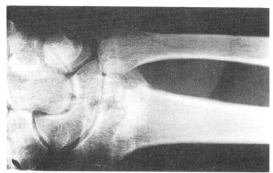

Fig. 2.21 Malunion of a Colles' fracture. Anteroposterior radiograph showing impaction and relative lengthening of the ulna with subluxation of the distal radio-ulnar joint.

1. Dorsal angulation and displacement (Fig. 2.20).
2. Simple impaction of the radial fracture, giving a relative lengthening of the ulna (Fig. 2.21).
3. Combinations of 1. and 2.

TREATMENT

The best way to prevent malunion is to adequately reduce the fracture and to hold the reduction by immobilizing the fracture in dorsal and radial slabs in palmar flexion and ulnar deviation (Fig. 2.22). In some cases where there is comminution and severe crushing of the cancellous bone external fixation or crossed Kirschner wires may be necessary.

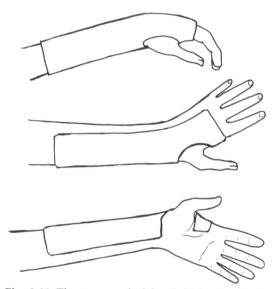

Fig. 2.22 The types of slabs (which should be applied over padding) for a Colles' fracture.

Once malunion is established correction is necessary only if the function is impaired or the result is cosmetically unacceptable. Remember most of these patients are elderly and are less likely to have functional disability or to worry about the cosmetic result.

Correction of malunion where there is dorsal angulation requires an osteotomy of the distal radius and often the insertion of a bone graft (Fig. 2.23).

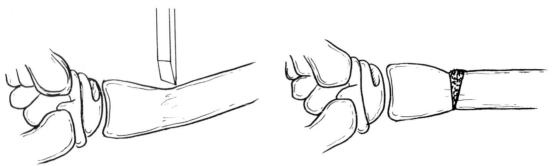

Fig. 2.23 Operative correction from the dorsal aspect of the radius with the insertion of a wedge of bone.

KEY POINTS

a. **A dorsal approach using a longitudinal incision on the ulnar side of the extensor pollicus longus.**
b. **The fracture site is the best place to do the osteotomy. The distal part containing the articular surface can be angled forward with an osteotome.**
c. **A bone graft should be placed in the gap. The reconstruction can then be held with two Kirschner wires or a small T-plate.**

KEY POINTS

a. **Shortening of the ulna is done easily though a short incision along the ulnar border. The amount to be removed should be calculated on the radiograph and marked on the bone with an osteotome.**
b. **The distal mark should be about a half a centimetre from the distal end of the ulna.**
c. **Drill a hole through the distal end of the ulna and up the shaft. Remove the small segment and insert a malleolar self-tapping lag screw and tighten the screw. The gap should close completely and the ulna will heal quickly.**

Correction of malunion with impaction of the radius and relative lengthening of the ulna can be achieved by either excision of the distal end of the ulna or by shortening of the ulna just proximal to the distal end (Fig. 2.24).

Combined lesions are managed by radial osteotomy and the insertion of a bone graft which corrects both the dorsal angulation and restores length.

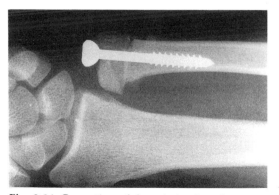

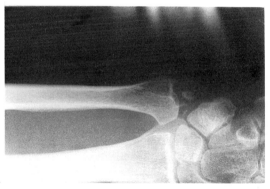

Fig. 2.24 Correction of the relative lengthening of the ulna by shortening and internal fixation with a screw. The screw will need to be removed later.

Fig. 2.25 An ununited fracture of the ulnar styloid. This is only rarely persistently painful.

(ii) Non union

The radial fracture always unites as it occurs at a site where the radius is largely cancellous. However the ulnar styloid process, which is often but not always fractured, commonly remains ununited (Fig. 2.25).

TREATMENT

Persistent symptoms such as local tenderness and pain on radial deviation are rare but do occur. When symptoms are severe and remain present after six months, local excision of the fragment is indicated. This operation is done through a short incision along the ulnar border taking care to avoid the dorsal branch of the ulnar nerve.

(iii) Carpal tunnel syndrome

This condition can follow a Colles' fracture and may come on acutely while the patient is in plaster but more commonly occurs after removal of the plaster and the resumption of activity. The reason for the development of this condition is that after a Colles' fracture that has displaced there is often physically less room in the carpal tunnel. The median nerve is compressed especially at night when there is no movement of the tendons to dispel oedema. This gives the classical symptoms of burning and tingling in the median nerve distribution which wake the patient and may be temporarily relieved by holding and shaking the hand towards the ground.

The diagnosis is a clinical one and the story is usually very clear. However if there is any doubt then electrical testing of the median nerve (EMG) will confirm a delay in nerve conduction.

TREATMENT

Division of the anterior carpal ligament through a short longitudinal incision in the palmar crease will permanently relieve the symptoms.

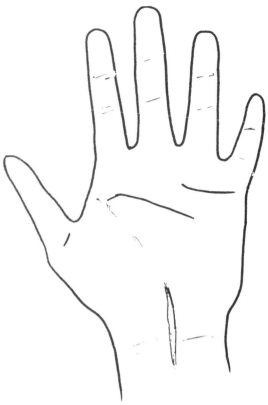

Fig. 2.26 The incision for carpal tunnel release. Note the anterior carpal ligament extends both proximally and distally and must be divided over its whole width.

KEY POINTS

a. The incision is deepened carefully through the muscular fibres of the flexor digitorum brevis (which often arise from the ligament) until the ligament is cut through at one point.

b. A dissector can then be placed over the median nerve and under the ligament to protect the nerve whilst the ligament is cut completely proximally and distally (Fig. 2.26).

c. Be sure the carpal tunnel is completely divided. You can insert your little finger to confirm complete division.

(iv) Tendon rupture

1. Extensor tendons

The extensor pollicus longus is the tendon which most frequently ruptures. This incident occurs about three weeks after the plaster is removed and the clinical picture is seen in Fig. 2.27. This patient has been asked to extend the thumbs of both hands. Rupture of the tendon occurs more frequently in the elderly but can occur at any age if there is a sharp projection of bone on which the tendon rubs.

TREATMENT

It is impossible to carry out direct repair since the proximal muscular end retracts and in any case the ends are shredded and there will not be sufficient length to allow repair.

One of a number of tendon transfers can be done:

Extensor indicis can be transferred as the motor and joined to the distal

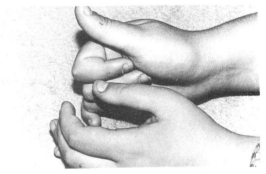

Fig. 2.27 Testing for the integrity of the extensor pollicus longus.

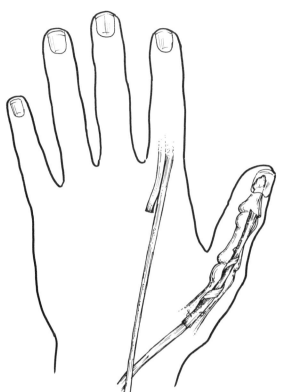

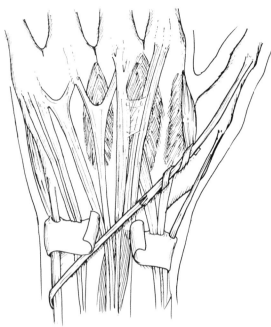

Fig. 2.29 Transfer of the flexor superficialis around the ulnar border to the extensor pollicus longus.

Fig. 2.28 Extensor indicis transfer to the extensor pollicus longus.

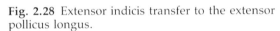

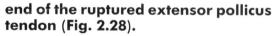

end of the ruptured extensor pollicus tendon (Fig. 2.28).

Flexor superficialis tendon from the ring finger can be divided at the base of the finger and brought around the ulnar side of the wrist and attached to the distal stump (Fig. 2.29). The palmaris longus may also be used in this way but may be absent and in any case is often too short.

Extensor carpi radialis longus can be used as the motor (this is my choice as the tendon is the right length and the muscle is powerful and seems to have enough excursion) (Fig. 2.30).

2. Flexor tendons

Rupture of one or more flexor tendons has been reported but is rare. The most common flexor tendon to rupture is the flexor pollicus longus. This is easily recognized by the patient being unable to flex the distal phalanx of the thumb (Fig. 2.31).

TREATMENT

Direct repair is not possible due to retraction and the poor state of the tendon at the site of rupture. A tendon transfer using the palmaris longus tendon, or the flexor superficialis tendon from the ring finger (Fig. 2.32) gives good results.

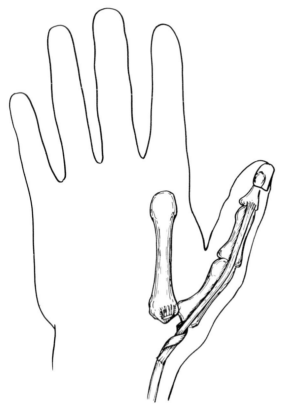

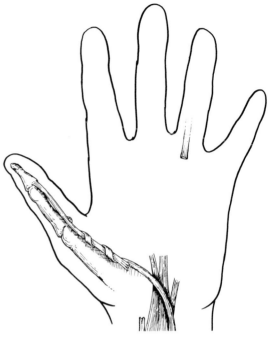

Fig. 2.32 Transfer of the flexor superficialis to the ring finger to the flexor pollicus longus.

Fig. 2.30 Transfer of the extensor carpi radialis to the extensor pollicus longus.

(v) Sudek's atrophy (Reflex sympathetic dystrophy)

This serious complication occurs rarely. It involves an adult patient who usually has suffered a fracture of the wrist (or ankle) or had an operation on a limb. The injury or operation is often quite a minor one. The patient tends to be an anxious nervous person. There is intense and often unduly prolonged pain, vasomotor disturbances and rapid development of trophic changes and loss of function.

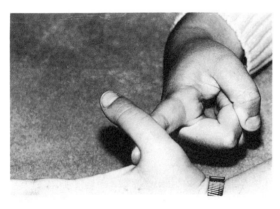

Fig. 2.31 Testing for the integrity of the flexor pollicus longus.

The symptoms are pain, swelling, pitting oedema, tenderness, bluish tinge to the skin, coldness, and shiny atrophic skin. The pain can be intense and burning and discourages movement. It is often aggravated by heat or touching the limb. Symptoms can last for weeks or even months and then gradually

The poor blood flow allows a low pH to develop and promotes localized demineralization of bone giving the unusual and diagnostic appearance of spotty demineralization of the bones. Because there is ischaemia in the tissues, fibrin becomes deposited and fibrosis of the tissues can cause permanent stiffness. Excessive sweating is caused by overstimulation of the sympathetic system.

TREATMENT

You will need the help of your physiotherapist, on a two or three times daily basis as the patient will require:

1. **Elevation of the limb.**
2. **Mobilization by active exercises under analgesia.**
3. **Avoidance of extreme heat or cold.**
4. **Sympathetic blocks and in some cases sympathectomy.**

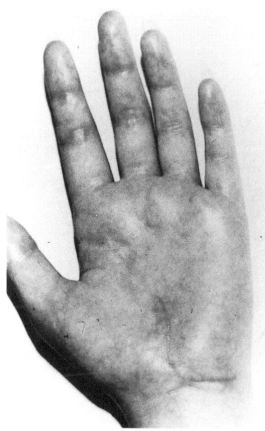

Fig. 2.33 Sudek's atrophy as it affects the hand.

subside leaving a hand or a foot which is stiff and cold and has an atrophic look with shiny skin and tapered fingers (Fig. 2.33). Not all cases progress to the full blown syndrome, especially if treatment is commenced early and pursued vigorously. A widespread disturbance of central autonomic regulation is generally considered responsible. The mechanism of the condition is thought to be due to vasospasm of the small arterioles giving poorly flowing blood in the arterioles and capillaries and this gives the blue appearance and the coldness of the affected part. The oedema is due to the outflow from the capillaries of plasma and fibrin.

Intravenous guanethidine has been used to achieve a chemical sympathetic block with good effect. It acts as a false transmitter and is taken up by sympathetic nerve endings and displaces norepinephrine (noradrenaline) from its storage sites. This block can last for several days after one injection.

Guanethidine is given intravenously in an exsanguinated limb using a similar technique to a Bier block for local anaesthesia. Warning: orthostatic hypotension, dizziness, somnolence and nausea can occur. Use only under expert supervision.

Epidural anaesthesia offers an alternative to lumbar sympathetic blocks in the lower limb and has the advantage of being able to be 'topped up' if an infusion catheter is used.

STELLATE BLOCK _____

Stellate block can be done as an out-patient procedure. The stellate ganglion lies in front of the transverse process of the seventh cervical vertebra, in front of the first rib, and posterior to the vertebral artery.

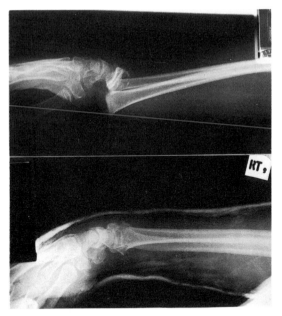

Fig. 2.34 Juvenile Colles' fracture. Note it is a Salter Harris type 2 epiphyseal fracture and usually the epiphyseal plate is undamaged.

With this anatomical position it is not surprising that this technique requires skill and the ability to handle possible complications (such as pneumothorax). I leave this block to my anaesthetist.

With a successful injection and blocking of the ganglion a Horner's syndrome, dryness of the hand and arm and a vasodilatation plus the relief of pain, are confirmatory signs that the injection is in the right place.

Having achieved the block the pain cycle is broken (sometimes only temporarily) and vigorous active exercises should be carried out. It may be necessary to repeat the block on several occasions. Each time a programme of intensive exercise should reduce the level of pain, swelling and stiffness. Persistent symptoms may warrant sympathectomy.

(b) Colles' fracture in juveniles

This fracture usually unites without problems, however occasionally we see:

1. Malunion;
2. Epiphyseal damage to the distal radial epiphysis.

Slight malunion is not infrequent as these fractures are often prone to re-displacing if the plaster gets loose quickly. Fortunately the child is usually young and the angulation can be accepted as there will be rapid moulding and correction. The closer a fracture is to the epiphysis and the younger the child, the more rapid and the more complete the correction (Fig. 2.34).

Epiphyseal damage is also rare, fortunately as the fracture usually is a Salter Harris type 2 injury with a sliver of metaphysis protecting the epiphysis. The various types of epiphyseal injuries are shown in Fig. 2.35 according to the classification devised by Salter and Harris.

When the epiphysis is damaged irregular growth or complete cessation of growth will occur. The bony bridge which crosses the epiphyseal plate can be peripheral or central. Depending on the type of bridge, the wrist joint will deform most commonly with relative overgrowth of the ulna, dislocation of the distal radio-ulnar joint and radial deviation of the hand (Fig. 2.36).

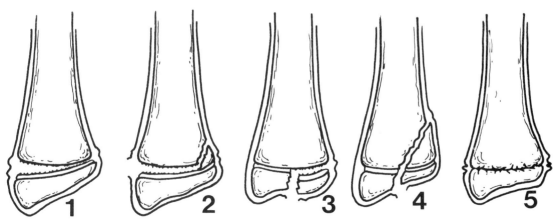

Fig. 2.35 Salter Harris classification of epiphyseal injuries. 1, Greenstick type; 2, juxta-epiphyseal with a piece of metaphysis; 3, trans-epiphyseal; 4, trans-epiphyseal extending into the metaphysis; 5, crushing of the epiphyseal plate.

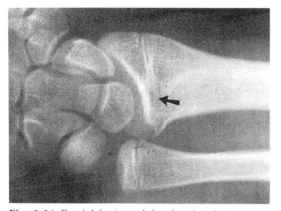

Fig. 2.36 Partial fusion of the distal radial epiphysis (arrow) with relative overgrowth of the ulna.

Where epiphyseal damage occurs it may be possible to:

1. Remove a bony bridge partially stopping epiphyseal growth and fill the space with fat or silastic (epiphyseolysis) (Fig. 2.37).
2. Either in combination with the above or separately do a corrective osteotomy to allow re-alignment of the joint surfaces.
3. Carry out an epiphyseodesis on the distal ulna and the remnants of the radial epiphysis to prevent further deformity when it is not possible to obtain further growth correction (Fig. 2.38).

TREATMENT

Mostly the damage to the epiphysis is done at the time of injury. Further damage should be avoided by:

1. non-violent reduction of the fracture.
2. avoidance of open reduction where possible in type 2 fractures.

KEY POINTS

Key points in epiphyseolysis

a. Operate early before there is much deformity.
b. Preoperatively obtain tomograms to determine the size and location of the bony bridge.
c. Using magnification (operating loupes or a microscope), locate the bony bridge and excise completely so that the

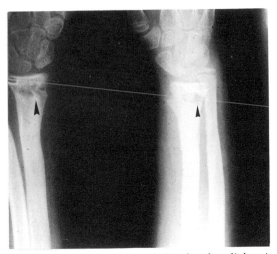

Fig. 2.37 Epiphyseolysis of the distal radial epiphysis.

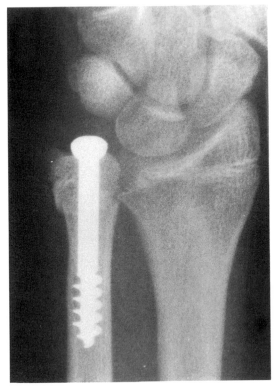

Fig. 2.38 Epiphyseodesis of the distal ulnar epiphysis.

epiphyseal plate is visible all around the bridge. The use of a dental pic and small burrs make it easier. You may also need radiographs during the procedure.

d. Insert some free fat or silastic into the defect.

KEY POINTS

Key points in corrective osteotomy

a. Correction should be done in the metaphysis 2–3 cm from the epiphysis.

b. The osteotomy that corrects the malalignment best is not an opening or closing wedge but one in which the apex of the triangle created by the opening wedge is moved far enough towards the centre of the bone to allow easy correction without leaving a large gap (Fig. 2.39).

c. The osteotomy can be held by smooth pins in the metaphysis and in the epiphysis. The pins can be attached to an external frame or incorporated in plaster.

KEY POINTS

Key points in epiphyseodesis

a. The easiest way to stop an epiphysis growing is to cut out a rectangular piece including metaphysis, epiphyseal plate and epiphysis.

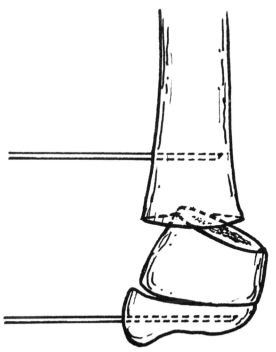

Fig. 2.39 Diagram of a translocation osteotomy.

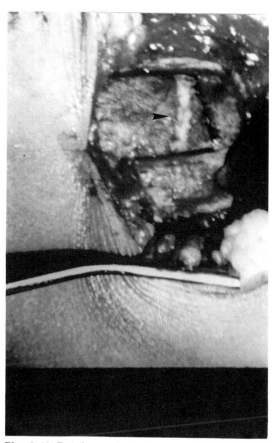

Fig. 2.40 Epiphyseodesis by reversing a bone plug which includes the epiphyseal line.

b. Through the bed of this rectangle curette out as much of the plate as is visible.
c. Now reverse the rectangular bone plug, so that the proximal end is inserted distally (Fig. 2.40).

(c) Scaphoid fractures

(i) Delayed union and non union

This is the most frequent problem associated with this fracture.

Delayed union is present if not united after 12 weeks, and non union if not united after 20 weeks.

TREATMENT

Both conditions warrant open reduction and internal fixation and if there is any gap, bone grafting. In cases such as sedentary workers, some non unions can be treated by soft tissue interposition at the fracture site.

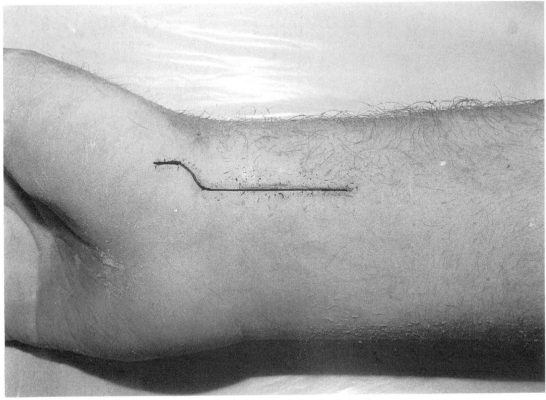

Fig. 2.41 The skin incision for the anterior approach to the scaphoid.

KEY POINTS

Key points in technique

a. An anterior incision 3 cm long lateral to the flexor carpi radialis tendon, with an S curve so that there is not a straight incision across the wrist joint (Fig. 2.41).

b. Deepen the incision through the lateral and posterior parts of the flexor carpi radialis tendon sheath, retract the tendon laterally, this protects the median nerve by having the tendon between you and the nerve. Working through the tendon sheath also keeps you clear of the radial artery (Fig. 2.42).

c. Open the wrist joint capsule and you are usually right at the fracture site.

d. A bone graft can be taken from the distal end of the radius which is cancellous, and internal fixation should be done using the Herbert screw (Fig. 2.43).

Always use a bone graft in non union, a wedge-shaped graft with an anterior base should be used.

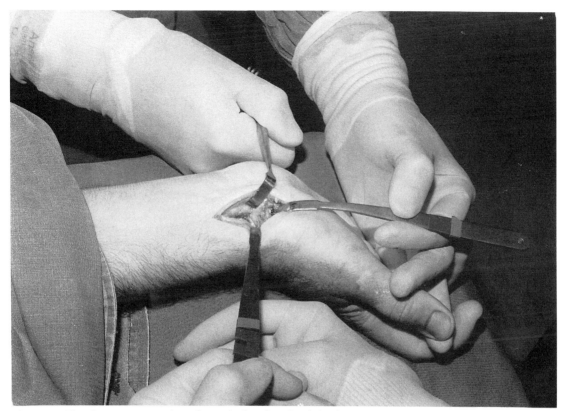

Fig. 2.42 The deeper approach is through the sheath of the flexor carpi radialis tendon which protects the median nerve and the radial artery.

e. **Occasionally where non union is established one choice of treatment can be local soft tissue interposition at the fracture site. This treatment,which leaves the scaphoid in two pieces prevents it from acting as a keystone in the carpal architecture. The operation is attributed to Bentzon and works quite well in sedentary workers.**

(ii) Traumatic arthritis

This condition can develop almost unnoticed after a fractured scaphoid is missed and present years later as an established arthritis after a trivial injury brings it to our attention (Fig. 2.44).

TREATMENT

This will vary according to the severity of pain and the damage to the joints. Simple immobilization may be enough to allow the wrist to settle. If it is not then the options are:

1. **Excision of the radial styloid process (Fig. 2.45).**
2. **Local arthrodesis (Fig. 2.46).**
3. **Arthrodesis of the wrist (Fig. 2.47).**
4. **Replacement arthroplasty of the scaphoid (Fig. 2.48).**

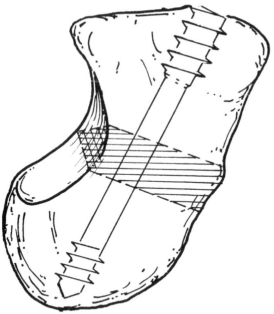

Fig. 2.43 Inserting a wedge based anteriorly restores the length and shape of the scaphoid as a 'keystone' in the wrist.

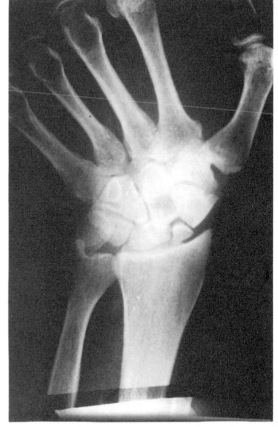

Fig. 2.44 Early arthritis 10 years after a fractured scaphoid.

KEY POINTS

1. **Radial styloidectomy is simple and effective for localized arthritis, a simple 3 cm lateral incision and an angled ostectomy of the styloid.**
2. **Local arthrodesis between the scaphoid and the radius or between the scaphoid, lunate and the radius is successful if these are the joints involved.**
   a. **Use a dorsal incision, retract tendons and nerves.**
   b. **Remove articular surfaces back to cancellous bone.**
   c. **Fit the bones together and pack in cancellous bone from the distal radius.**
   d. **Hold the bones together**

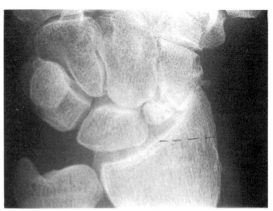

Fig. 2.45 The bone to be removed when excising the radial styloid.

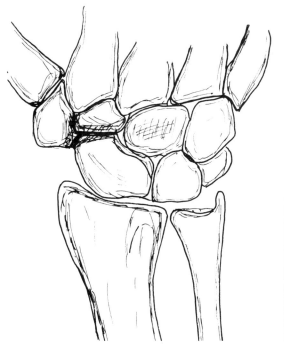

Fig. 2.46 Local arthrodesis of the scaphoid and its neighbours gives a tri-scaphoid. It is useful in local arthritis.

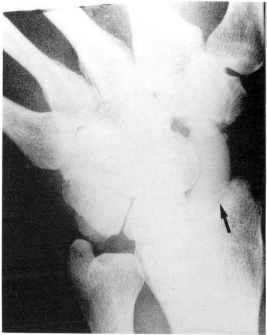

Fig. 2.48 Silastic replacement of the scaphoid. Obtaining stability of the implant is the problem.

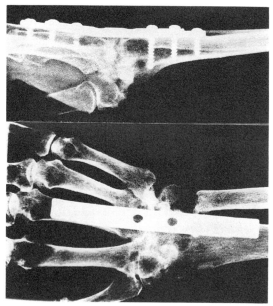

Fig. 2.47 Arthrodesis of the wrist using a plate and local bone grafts. The distal end of the ulna has been excised.

with Kirschner wires (Fig. 2.49).
3. **Arthrodesis of the wrist**
   This is a solution where the arthritis is generalized.
   a. Use a long dorsal incision, retracting the extensor tendons and dorsal veins.
   b. Excise the joint surfaces of the bones and pack bone chips in the spaces. This is easily done with an osteotome to excise articular surfaces and the use of local bone chips.

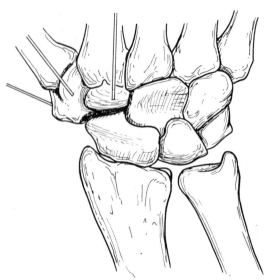

Fig. 2.49 Steps in the triscaphoid operation; excise the surfaces and fit together with Kirschner wires to hold in place.

c. **Mould a small Dynamic Compression Plate to fit onto the dorsal aspect of the distal radius and along the second or third metacarpal. Be sure that the wrist will not be held in ulnar or radial deviation.**
d. **Screw this into place providing firm fixation without the need for external support (Fig. 2.47).**
4. **Scaphoid replacement arthroplasty**
    This is not used frequently.
    a. **Dorsal and radial incision, incise the capsule lateral to the extensor carpi radialis longus and retract the extensor pollicus longus, preserve the capsule.**

b. **Remove the scaphoid and use test prostheses to determine the size of the prosthetic replacement.**
c. **Drill a hole in the trapezium for the stem of the prosthesis and insert and lock in the implant. Securely repair the capsule.**
d. **Immobilize the wrist for a few weeks to allow the capsule to repair and then gently mobilize.**

2.2 FOREARM BONES

2.2.1 RADIUS AND ULNA

(a) Galeazzi fracture

This is a fracture of the radius in its distal half and the dislocation of the distal end of the ulna (Fig. 2.50). If there is any degree of malunion then the distal radio-ulnar joint will be disrupted.

It is not uncommon for this joint to remain dislocated if angulation is accepted at the radial fracture.

TREATMENT

Even if the fracture is neglected there may still be an opportunity to carry out open reduction of the radius with internal fixation, and the dislocated ulna head may be relocated. However in the very late case it may not be possible to restore full length to the radius.

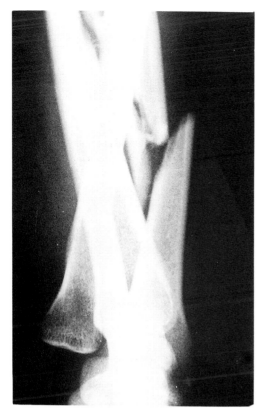
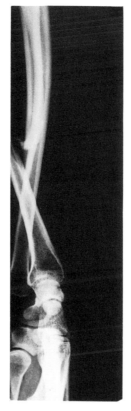
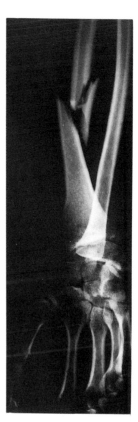

Fig. 2.50 Galeazzi fracture. Note the dislocation of the distal radio-ulnar joint.

```
┌─── KEY POINTS ──────────────┐
```
KEY POINTS

a. **Always restore length and alignment of the radius, if possible and internally fix with compression techniques.**

b. **If the distal radio-ulnar joint is dislocated, await union of the fractured radius and then either shorten the ulna or excise the head of the ulna.**

c. **The techniques for ulnar shortening and excision of the distal ulna have already been detailed above, under complications of Colles' fracture (Fig. 2.24).**

(b) Radius and ulna in adults

(i) Malunion

This is the most frequent complication in this area. The problem can be avoided with care:

1. Always try for end to end apposition where closed reduction is used;
2. Angulation in mid shaft fractures is not acceptable;
3. Plaster immobilization must be in a long arm cast in mid position for upper and middle third fractures and in full supination for distal third fractures;
4. Unless satisfactory position is obtained open reduction, compression plating and bone grafting should be carried out;

5. The treatment of choice in adults for all displaced fractures is compression plating and bone grafting.

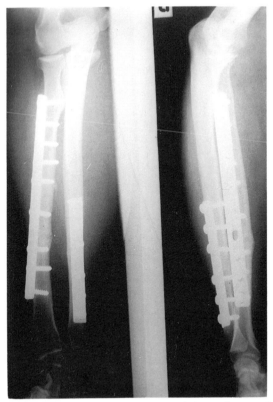

Fig. 2.51 Compression plating of the radius and ulna.

KEY POINTS

Key points in compression plating and bone grafting the radius and ulna (Fig. 2.51).

a. **Always use a separate incision for the radius and ulna (to avoid cross union).**
b. **Expose the easier fracture (less comminuted) first, and hold it reduced as far as possible with a plate and clamps. Do not screw in place at this stage.**
c. **Expose the other bone through a separate incision and reduce. You may need to adjust the first reduction. Both should be perfect before the easier of the fractures is plated and screwed under compression. The plates must be long enough, preferably three holes on each side of the fracture (Fig. 2.52).**
d. **I routinely add a bone graft. The graft can be taken from the opposite iliac crest. (Some surgeons may disagree but I am certain this is worthwhile as it will prevent delayed and non union).**

TREATMENT OF MALUNION

Deformity can be corrected by osteotomy and plating, together with bone grafting (Fig. 2.53).

KEY POINTS

a. **Always carry out the correction at the site of the deformity.**
b. **Be careful not to burn the bone with a saw cut. Use drill holes and an osteotome.**
c. **Fixation must be secure, always add a bone graft.**
d. **Always try for but do not expect full return of function.**

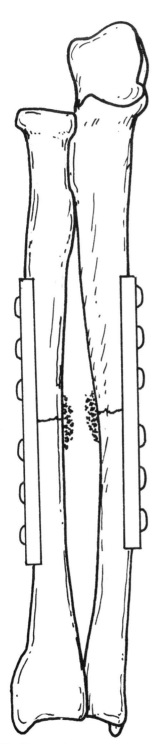

Fig. 2.52 Ideally the plates should be long enough to allow three screws on each side of the fracture.

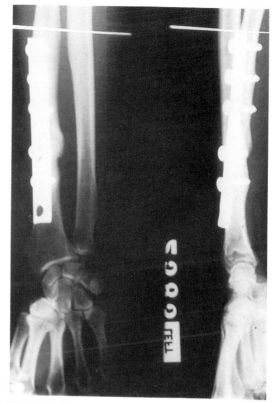

Fig. 2.53 Correction of a malunited radius by osteotomy and plating.

(ii) Cross union

Fortunately this is not common. It tends to occur when there is extensive soft tissue injury and it can follow open reduction and internal fixation when this is done through a single incision. What occurs is basically an ossification of the fracture or operation haematoma. The effect is to lock the forearm and prevent rotary movement (Fig. 2.54).

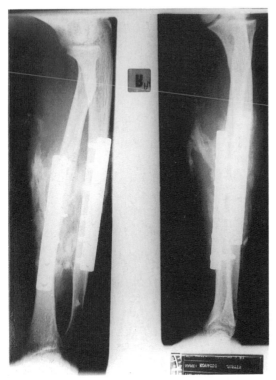

Fig. 2.54 Cross union of a fractured radius and ulna. There will be no pronation and supination.

TREATMENT

Where the cross union is widespread it is unlikely that excision will be successful. Small areas can be excised taking great care with haemostasis and using a silastic insert to try and keep the bones from re-uniting. Very often the poor result is associated with the ossification of the interosseous membrane as well as the bony bridge between the radius and ulna.

(iii) Delayed union and non union (see also section 1.2.2)

Delayed union is said to have occurred when a fracture of the forearm has not united in twelve weeks (Fig. 2.55). Since the treatment is similar it will be discussed under non union which is said to have occurred (for practical purposes) when fractures of both bones of the forearm have not united in twenty weeks (Fig. 2.56).

KEY POINTS

a. **Where both bones of the forearm are fractured you must restore stability to the rectangle (Fig. 2.57). Restore the length of both the radius and ulna and see that the proximal and distal radio–ulnar joints are reduced. The best way to do this in adults is to carry out open reduction and internal fixation using compression techniques.**

b. **In all cases of delayed union, non union, and all adult forearm fractures an extensive bone graft needs to be used. This is best removed from the inner table of the iliac crest (Fig. 1.26). Some surgeons may disagree with the routine use of a bone graft in adult fractures undergoing open reduction and plating. I must say I have never been sorry I bone grafted a forearm, but I have met may others who have been sorry they did not.**

c. **Semitubular plates are not strong enough in adults, use a AO/ASIF DCP plate and be sure that the plate is long enough. I prefer to have three holes above and three below the fracture site.**

d. **Where a short plate has been used and has come loose, try to avoid using the same screw holes and use a considerably longer plate.**

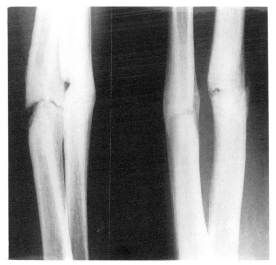

Fig. 2.55 Delayed union of a fractured forearm; radiographs taken at 16 and 26 weeks.

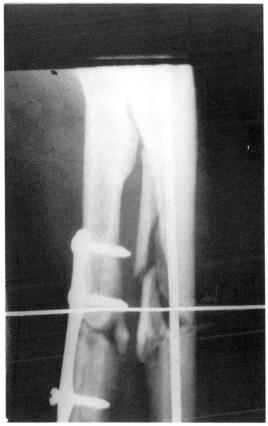

Fig. 2.56 Non union of a fractured radius and ulna at twenty weeks. The fractures are held apart by the internal fixation.

(c) Radius and ulna in children

Alignment problems that arise in forearm fractures are similar in adults and children, however children have the ability to mould and remodel bone, so that we can accept some angulation, some displacement and even some rotary displacement.

Important factors

1. Age of the child, below the age of eight most deformities will correct themselves within one to two years.
2. Proximity to the epiphysis, the closer to the epiphysis the quicker and more complete the recovery.
3. Rotary deformity recovers less fully and often leaves limited pronation and supination especially over the age of eight.

TREATMENT

In the older child correction of the deformity at the fracture sites using the technique of multiple drill holes and osteoclasis (breaking the bone) is recommended (Fig. 2.58).

(d) Monteggia fracture

This is a common and complicated fracture in children and adults. The most frequent problem is that one component of the fracture is

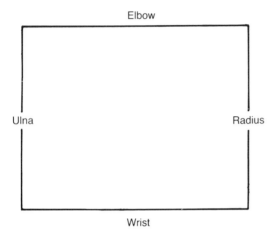

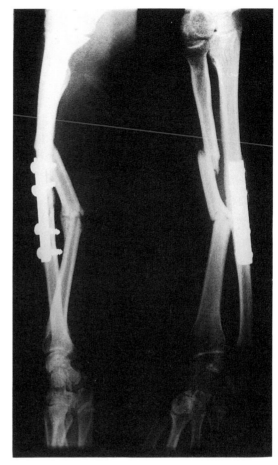

Fig. 2.57 The rectangle concept in forearm fractures. In the radiograph note that the length of the ulna has been restored by plating but the radius is in pieces and malaligned. The distal end of the ulna must be dislocated.

not recognized. There are two breaks in the rectangle (Fig. 2.57), a fracture of the ulna usually in the proximal half and a dislocation of the head of the radius. The dislocation of the head of the radius can be overlooked by the inexperienced.

Remember

(a) If the head of the radius is dislocated there must be a fracture of the ulna (Fig. 2.59).
(b) If there is a displaced fracture of the ulna make sure you see the elbow and wrist joints as there must be another fracture or dislocation present in the radial axis.

Malunion of Monteggia practure

In children some angulation of the ulnar fragment can be accepted as it will remodel provided the radial head is reduced and stays reduced. There will be remarkably little restriction of pronation and supination.

In adults do not accept poor position. Carry out open reduction and compression plating of the ulna and then the radial head dislocation is easy to control.

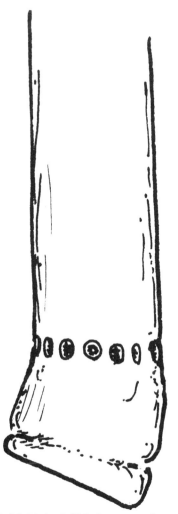

Fig. 2.58 Multiple drill holes to weaken the bone and allow osteoclasis.

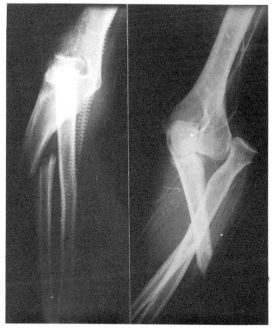

Fig. 2.59 Monteggia fracture. Note the dislocated head of the radius.

TREATMENT

Osteotomize the ulna at the old fracture site to correct the deformity and allow lengthening of the ulna and reposition the head of the radius. This is best done in two stages. The radial head should be dissected free and a trial reduction done. If this works then an osteotomy of the ulna can be done just distal to the proximal radio-ulnar notch. A grossly distorted and oversized head of the radius cannot be reduced.

KEY POINTS

a. **Use a Boyd incision (posterolateral lifting aside the anconeus and exposing the posterior aspect of the head of the radius) (Fig. 2.60).**
b. **Clear out the normal area for the head of the radius which is full of capsular and annular ligament remnants and fibrous tissue.**
c. **Osteotomize the ulna at the peak of the deformity and straighten the bone allowing the ulna to lengthen.**
d. **When the head of the radius is relocated, plate the ulna and bone graft the defect in the ulna.**
e. **Fashion a new annular ligament for the head of the radius from the central slip of the triceps (Fig. 2.61).**

2.2.2 AROUND THE ELBOW JOINT

(a) Neck and head of radius

(i) Malunion in children

In children fractures of the neck of the radius are common. The displacement of the fracture varies from nil to the head being totally displaced from the neck (Fig. 2.62). As always in children, there will be considerable recovery due to moulding and growth. The critical angle allowable seems to be 30 degrees of angulation. Beyond this point there will be loss of pronation and supination and some loss of flexion and extension of the elbow.

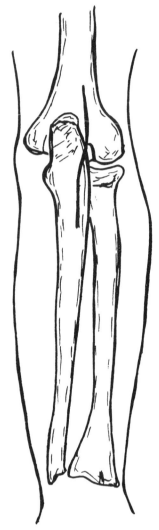

Fig. 2.60 The Boyd incision allows access to the head of the radius and the back of the elbow joint.

TREATMENT

The deformity can be corrected by osteotomy of the neck of the radius. Do not excise the head of the radius in children as a cubitus valgus deformity will result and later an ulnar palsy.

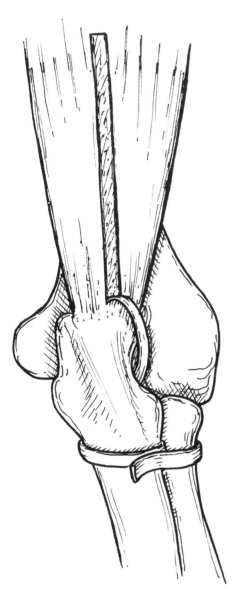

Fig. 2.61 Use a strip of the triceps tendon to fashion a new annular ligament to contain the head of the radius.

KEY POINTS

a. In all operations on the head of the radius a lateral incision can be used but do not extend this distally or the posterior inter-osseus branch of the radial nerve will be in danger (Fig. 2.63).
b. Drill two holes through the neck of the radius and then break the neck. Use an osteotome to first cut partly into the neck, joining the two holes and then to incompletely fracture the neck and lever it straight.
c. If the osteotomy is done carefully it will be stable. If unstable a Kirschner wire may be used to stabilize the head in the corrected position.

(ii) Fractures of the head of the radius in adults

These fractures are common and generally the treatment is satisfactory. Problems arise because:

1. This is an intra-articular fracture which occurs when a force is transmitted up the shaft of the radius to the head and to the corresponding area of the humerus, the capitellum.
2. There is often significant damage to the articular surface of the capitellum and the head of the radius in addition to the fracture.

There may be loss of extension of the elbow and loss of pronation and supination of the forearm.

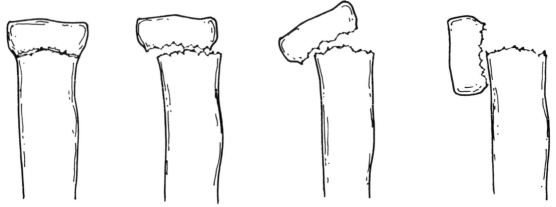

Fig. 2.62 Examples of the differing degrees of angulation and displacement of fractures of the neck of the radius.

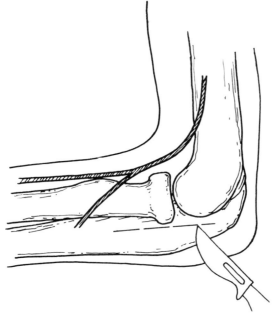

Fig. 2.63 The danger to the posterior interosseous branch of the radial nerve with a lateral incision that extends distally can be seen.

TREATMENT

Where there is evidence of severe damage to the joint surfaces excision of the head of the radius will improve the range of movement and lessen pain. Full movement is rarely obtained.

KEY POINTS

a. Use a lateral incision, do not extend the incision distally more than 4 cm distal to the lateral epicondyle or you will endanger the posterior interosseous nerve (Fig. 2.63).
b. Excise the head using a sharp osteotome cutting through the neck (Fig. 2.64).
c. Your assistant at the operation should initially hold the forearm in mid pronation and later fully pronate and supinate to allow you to cut through the neck cleanly.
d. Excision of the head of the radius does not leave the patient with a normal elbow. Some restriction of movement is the rule and about 5% of patients develop wrist symptoms due to the distal end of the ulna subluxing. Excision of the radial head should be avoided in heavy manual workers.

(iii) Malunion

Fractures of the head of the radius in adults tend to go through the head rather than the neck. Often a segment of the head is displaced and the articular surface then has a step.

TREATMENT

It is best to openly reduce these fractures and restore the articular surface. If this is not done initially and there is continuing pain and restriction of movement then the radial head should be excised.

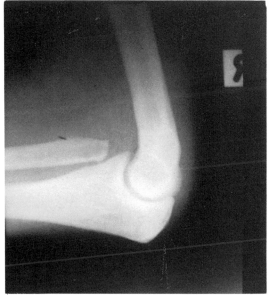

Fig. 2.64 Lateral radiograph after excision of the head of the radius.

KEY POINTS

a. **Use a lateral incision, do not extend the incision distally more than 4 cm distal to the lateral epicondyle or you will endanger the posterior interosseous nerve (Fig. 2.63).**
b. **Under direct vision reduce the fracture and hold temporarily with a Kirschner wire. Internal fixation using a Herbert Screw is advised as the head of the screw is buried and does not need removal (Fig. 2.65).**

(b) The olecranon

(i) Non union

The triceps tendon is inserted into the olecranon so that reduction and fixation of frac-

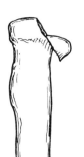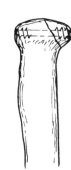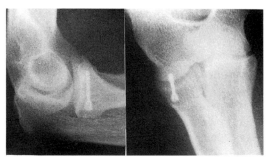

Fig. 2.65 The Herbert compression screw is ideal for holding fractures of the head of the radius.

tures of the olecranon need to withstand the pull of this powerful muscular force. Unless a fracture is undisplaced simple plaster immobilization is seldom good treatment. Bony union will occur if the fragments are well reduced and adequately fixed. Fibrous union may on occasions be painless and allow full function of the elbow especially if the fragment of olecranon is small.

TREATMENT

1. **Small fragments that do not involve the articular surface can be excised and the triceps insertion sutured.**
2. **Larger fragments and particularly those that involve the articular surface, need open reduction and internal fixation. Any gaps that are present due to comminution should be filled with bone graft.**

KEY POINTS

a. **Tension band wiring (Fig. 2.66) is the technique of choice as the fracture can be rigidly fixed and held without the need for plaster.**
b. **Use two parallel Kirschner wires and a figure of eight stainless steel wire which loops through a hole which is as far from the fracture as the fracture is from the olecranon tip. I use a No. 8 sternal wire which comes on an atraumatic needle, and that simplifies threading the wire through the hole.**
c. **Bend the ends of the wires to a U shape and drive them into the olecranon. Try to bury the knot of the stainless steel wire.**

d. **A lag screw can also be used but care needs to be taken to see that the threads of the screw do not cross the fracture line and hold the fracture apart (Fig. 2.67).**
e. **Use a bone graft to fill any gaps.**
f. **See that the fracture is accurately reduced as it is an intra-articular fracture.**

(ii) Removal of implants

Tension band wiring at the olecranon or the use of a lag screw often creates a problem as the screw can back out and become prominent, and the wires used in the tension band technique are subcutaneous and can cause discomfort when the patient leans on the elbow.

TREATMENT

Remove the implants when the fracture is solidly united, usually six to twelve months after open reduction.

KEY POINTS

a. **Remove the straight Kirschner wires through small incisions over the point of the elbow. They are easily located and removed.**
b. **Cut the continuous wire just distal to the knot, grasp the knot and pull out all the wire with strong pliers.**

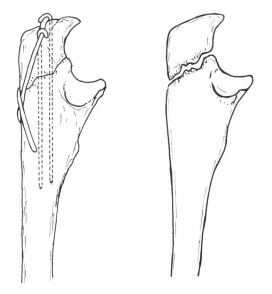

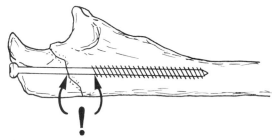

Fig. 2.67 Lag screw fixation of an olecranon fracture. Note, the threads must not cross the fracture line.

2.3 HUMERUS

2.3.1 CONDYLAR AND SUPRACONDYLAR IN CHILDREN

(a) Medial epicondyle

The medial epicondyle exists as a separate epiphysis from the age of five and fuses to the humerus at the age of fourteen. Between these ages you must look for the epiphysis in all radiographs of the elbow. If in doubt then take a radiograph of the other elbow for comparison. The epicondyle is commonly avulsed (Fig. 2.68) by the pull of the flexor digitorum and flexor carpi ulnaris which arise from a common origin on the medial epicondyle.

It can be:

1. Simply separated or avulsed with a bony fragment (Fig. 2.68).
2. Part of a fracture dislocation, the elbow is dislocated and the medial epicondyle is trapped in the joint (Fig. 2.69).
3. Below the age of five the cartilaginous medial epicondyle can very rarely be avulsed and catch in the elbow joint in a dislocation and prevent reduction.

Both require reduction and fixation of the fracture (Fig. 2.70).

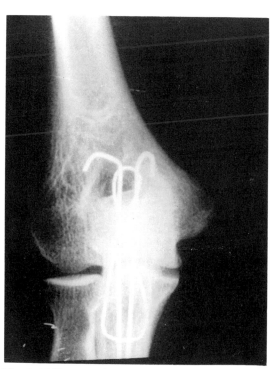

Fig. 2.66 Tension band wiring for a fracture of the olecranon. Note that this is an intra-articular fracture.

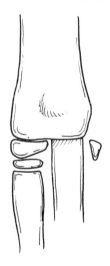

be done as a delayed procedure in neglected cases but there may be some difficulty in re-positioning the fragment in its bed.

KEY POINTS

a. **Use a medial incision being careful of the ulnar nerve (Fig. 2.71).**
b. **Identify the ulnar nerve and protect it. Transpose the nerve if it is running across the fracture line.**
c. **Pin the epicondyle in place with two Kirschner wires and bend the ends of the wires. You can use a screw in an older child as the epiphysis closes at the age of fifteen and there is no deformity if it closes a few years earlier.**

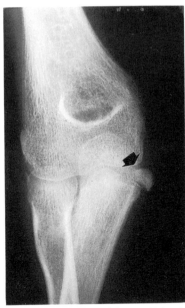

Established non union leaves the patient with some medial instability and pain over the medial epicondyle. The epicondyle can be fused to the humerus if the symptoms warrant intervention.

Fig. 2.68 Simple avulsion of the medial epicondyle.

(ii) Ulnar nerve injury

The ulnar nerve runs behind the medial epicondyle and is in danger at the time of injury, and during operative treatment (Fig. 2.72).

Preoperatively if there is any anaesthesia or hypoaesthesia then it is important to transpose the ulnar nerve.

(i) Non union

The pull of the flexor muscles means that vir-tually all these fractures displace. Displaced fractures will not proceed to bony union. Re-duction and fixation are necessary. This can

---

KEY POINTS

a. **This will be part of the open reduction and fixation of the epicondyle (see above).**
b. **The ulnar nerve is located in its groove and dissected free**

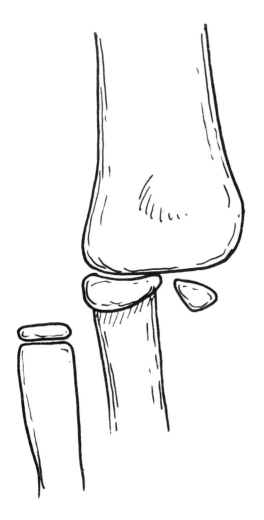

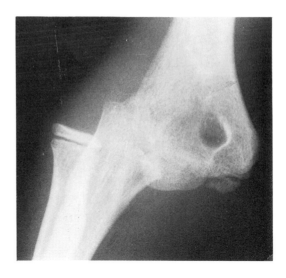

Fig. 2.69 Dislocation of the elbow with the epicondyle in the joint.

leaving the nerve covered with soft tissue as far as possible.

c. **Free the nerve so that it can lie anteriorly without tension. Be particularly careful that a sharp edge of fascia does not cut into the nerve proximally or distally.**

d. **Make a loose soft tissue sling to hold the nerve in its new home anteriorly.**

(b) Medial condyle

These fractures are rare injuries in childhood, but are important as they involve the trochlea and any malalignment will interfere with elbow function. Displaced fractures must be treated by open reduction and fixation (Fig. 2.73). Most fractures displace due to the pull of the flexor muscles.

Neglected fractures with displacement should be openly reduced and the fracture site cleaned out and reduction and pinning

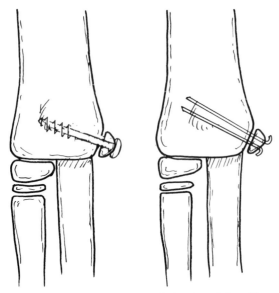

Fig. 2.70 Fixation of the medial epicondyle with a screw or wires.

The complications are:

carried out in much the same way as discussed above for fractures of the medial epicondyle.

(c) Lateral condyle

Fractures of the lateral condyle of the humerus occur with a fall on the outstretched hand when the elbow is extended. They usually displace and unless reduced leave a step in the joint. Very often the displacement is quite marked and the piece not only moves laterally but also rotates (Fig. 2.74).

Ideal treatment is reduction through a lateral incision and fixation with diverging Kirschner wires with their ends bent over (Fig. 2.75(a) and (b)).

Neglected fractures result in:

1. non union of the lateral condyle
2. valgus angulation at the elbow
3. poor elbow function
4. delayed (tardy) ulnar palsy

Other problems include the following.

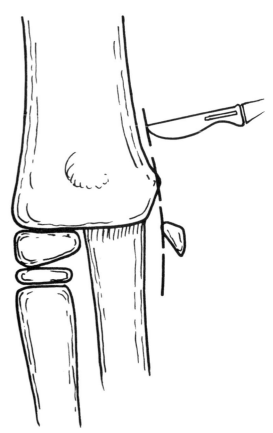

Fig. 2.71 The incision for pinning or screwing the medial epicondyle is just anterior to the medial supracondylar ridge.

(i) Premature fusion of the epiphysis

This can occur after the fracture and often all the epiphyses fuse giving no significant deformity. If only the lateral epiphysis fuses then a cubitus valgus can occur. It usually is mild and requires no treatment.

(ii) Avascular necrosis

Operative treatment of fractures of the lateral humeral condyle has its hazards and avascular necrosis is the most serious. It occurs when the soft tissue attachments to the lateral condyle are stripped too much thus

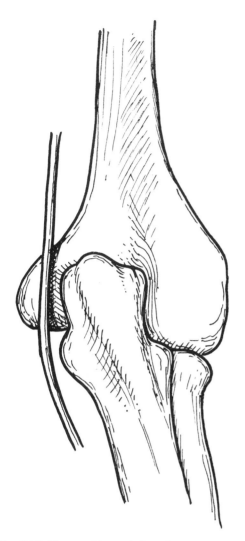

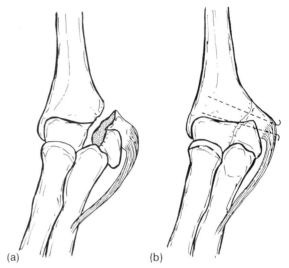

Fig. 2.73 (a) Displaced fracture of the medial condyle; (b) reduction and fixation is essential as there is always some rotation.

Fig. 2.72 The position of the ulnar nerve is just behind the medial epicondyle.

compromising the blood supply. There is no treatment except to correct any residual deformity.

TREATMENT

Delayed reduction is still worthwhile for some months after this injury as

although the elbow function is compromised and some loss of mobility is inevitable, you may prevent valgus deformity (Fig. 2.76). Beware of dissecting the lateral condyle too freely as avascular necrosis can result.

Once valgus deformity has occurred it will increase and there will be abnormal growth of the trochlea. When the varus increases ulnar nerve symptoms will develop due to stretching.

A varus osteotomy of the humerus will correct the angulation and release the traction on the ulnar nerve.

There are two types of osteotomy:

1. For those fractures that were due to a Salter Harris type 4 epiphyseal injury (Fig. 2.35) a closing wedge osteotomy is best.

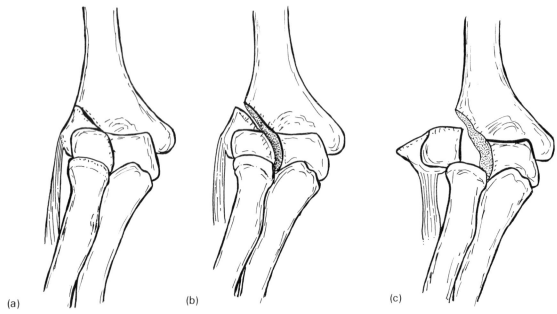

(a)   (b)   (c)

Fig. 2.74 (a), (b), and (c) Fractures of the lateral condyle can displace and often rotate.

KEY POINTS

a. **Use a medial incision from the medial epicondyle up the supracondylar ridge.**

b. **Transpose the ulnar nerve anteriorly (see section 2.3.1 (a) (ii)).**

c. **Remove a predetermined wedge with its base medially. The base should be wide enough to allow full correction of the angle of the elbow. Trace the outline of the radiograph with the humerus in the anatomical position, draw in the vertical axis and measure the deviation from this axis. This will give you the angle of the wedge, you can then work out the length of the base (Fig. 2.77).**

d. **Internally fix the osteotomized humerus with a plate and screws (Fig. 2.78).**

---

2. For those fractures of the lateral condyle that are Salter Harris type 2 epiphyseal injury (Fig. 2.35), a translocation osteotomy is best (Fig. 2.79).

KEY POINTS

a. **Through a medial incison transpose the ulnar nerve anteriorly as described above.**

b. **Through a lateral incision do a transverse osteotomy in the supracondylar region.**

c. **Displace the medial cortex laterally and rotate to correct both the angulation and alignment. Internally fix with one or two screws.**

(d) Supracondylar in children

This fracture is common at about the age of six and presents many challenges and problems.

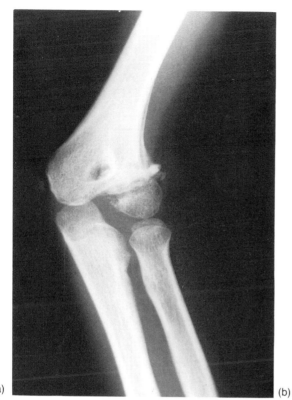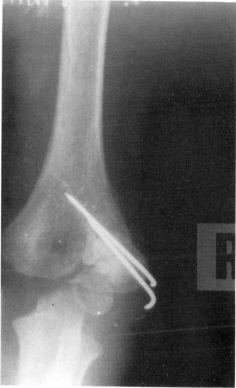

(a)   (b)

Fig. 2.75 (a) and (b) Accurate reduction and fixation are essential.

Amongst the complications are:

Vascular problems – immediate
Vascular problems – Volkmann's ischaemia
Volkmann's contracture
Difficulties in reduction
Redisplacement
Malunion
Nerve injuries
Myositis ossificans
Stiffness of the elbow

(i) Vascular problems – immediate

The six year old child with a grossly swollen and distorted elbow joint with a painful pallid hand and no radial pulse or capillary return represents a surgical emergency.

Figure 2.80 shows what often happens to the brachial artery in this injury. It is surprising in fact that there are so few cases of vascular problems as the brachial artery is only separated from the sharp edge of the proximal fragment by a thin sheet of the brachialis muscle. This muscle is usually torn when there is significant displacement.

TREATMENT

1. **Give some analgesia to the child and with traction straighten the fracture. This will often relieve the pressure on the brachial artery and the circulation will improve.**
2. **Make arrangements for anaesthesia and reduction of the fracture.**

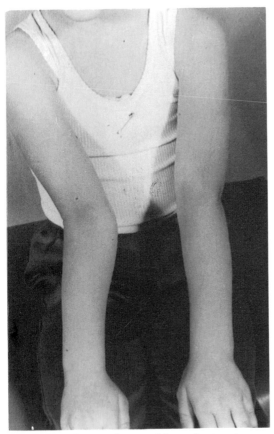

Fig. 2.76 Cubitus valgus and loss of extension are inevitable if the displaced fracture of the lateral condyle is not reduced.

Proceed with this as a matter of urgency as the longer the forearm muscles and nerves are without blood supply the worse the outlook.

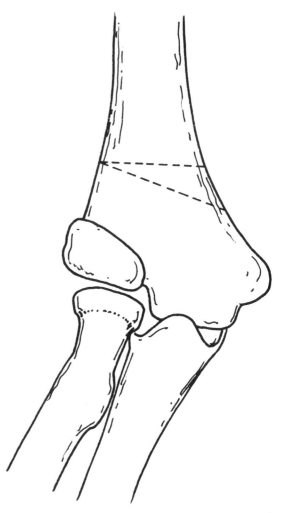

Fig. 2.77 Closing wedge osteotomy for a neglected displaced fracture of the lateral condyle of the humerus.

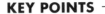

--- KEY POINTS ---

a. **Reduction of the displacement is carried out by traction, moving the displaced distal fragment back into alignment and then pushing the distal fragment anteriorly before**

flexing the elbow (Fig. 2.81, see also Fig. 2.91 (a), (b) and (c)).
b. **The elbow is now flexed slightly and you may need to wait a few minutes for the circulation to return. If it does return as evidenced by the return of capillary flow to the nail bed and perhaps the radial pulse,**

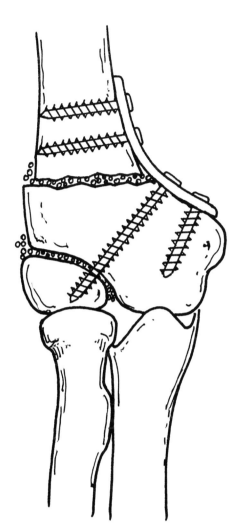

Fig. 2.78 After the osteotomy in Fig. 2.77 the reduction can be held by a plate and screws.

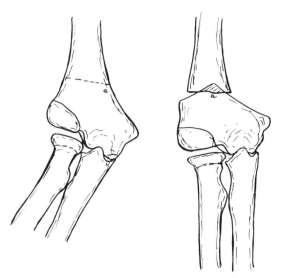

Fig. 2.79 Diagrams of a suitable translocation osteotomy of the distal humerus.

then a decision can be made regarding immobilization.

c. There is always gross swelling in the soft tissues in these cases and immobilization in plaster will need to be in flexion to only 90° or less otherwise the circulation will again be compromised.

d. When there is gross swelling it is better to put the child in

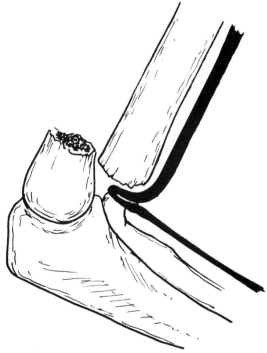

Fig. 2.80 The brachial artery can be caught over the jagged proximal end of the humerus.

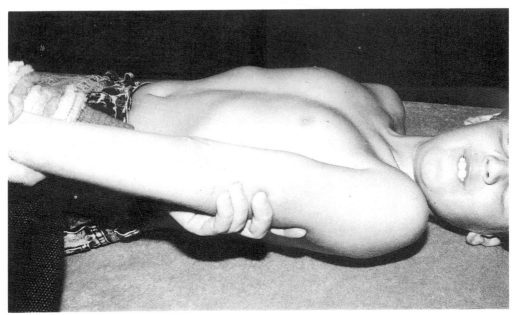

Fig. 2.81 Initial steps in reduction of a supracondylar fracture. The distal fragment and the shaft are aligned by traction and direct lateral or medial pressure.

overhead traction with a screw in the upper third of the ulna with the forearm supported in a sling (Fig. 2.82).

e. As an alternative Dunlop or other types of skin traction (Fig. 2.83) can be used until the swelling goes down and the situation stabilizes.

f. If the circulation does not return in a few minutes arrangements should proceed to explore the artery and to internally fix the fracture.

g. The artery is best explored through a Z shaped incision in the cubital fossa. The vessel may be impaled and stretched, compressed, or be partially or completely torn by the proximal fragment which can be razor sharp. In my series of 600 supracondylar fractures there were four acute vascular problems. All of these were due to the vessel being impaled on the sharp edge of the proximal fragment. All recovered without invasive vascular surgery, but spasm of the vessel took several minutes to disappear. Bathing the vessel with papaverine or local anaesthetic appeared to make no difference. Be prepared to excise and graft a damaged segment if necessary.

h. The easiest way to hold the fracture after open reduction is with crossed Kirschner wires inserted through the medial and lateral condyles posteriorly (Fig. 2.84). Be careful of the ulnar nerve on the medial side.

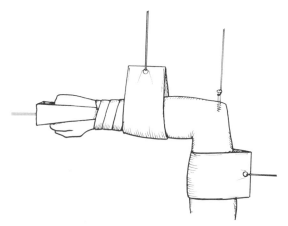

Fig. 2.82 Skeletal traction for a supracondylar fracture.

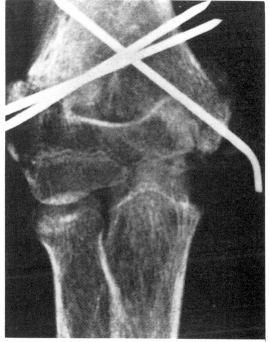

Fig. 2.84 Supracondylar fracture of the humerus held in good position with crossed Kirschner wires.

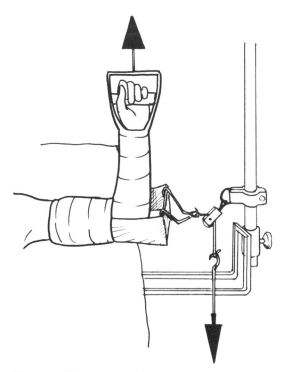

Fig. 2.83 Skin traction for a supracondylar fracture.

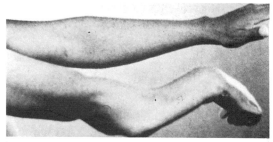

Fig. 2.85 The forearm deformity after a severe Volkman's ischaemic contracture.

(ii) Vascular problems – Volkmann's ischaemia

The price of failure to recognize and prevent this complication is disaster. There can be no more serious problem than a child whose fracture was reduced well, but ends up with a

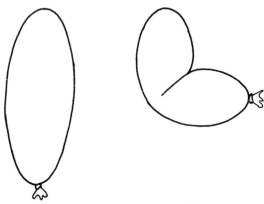

Fig. 2.86 The swollen elbow is like a sausage shaped balloon. Note where the pressure and indentation occurs when you flex the balloon.

Volkmann's ischaemia in the forearm and hand (Fig. 2.85).

The symptoms and signs are clear and definite:

1. Severe pain in the forearm muscles that are being starved of blood. (This pain will later disappear as all sensation is lost.)
2. Limitation of finger movement which is extremely painful.
3. Purple discolouration of the hand with prominent veins.
4. Initial paraesthesia followed by loss of sensation.
5. Loss of radial pulse and later loss of capillary return.
6. Finally pallor, anaesthesia and paralysis.

Volkmann's ischaemic necrosis occurs when the blood supply to the forearm muscles, nerves and skin are compromised by the artery being compressed at the elbow or in the forearm. This can follow the application of a full cast around the elbow or too much flexion of a very swollen elbow (Fig. 2.86). Mild swelling does not affect the vasculature (Fig. 2.87) but with an arm in a full cast that is too tight, the swelling, tight fascia and tight cast stop the circulation (Fig. 2.88).

Depending on the severity of the lesion

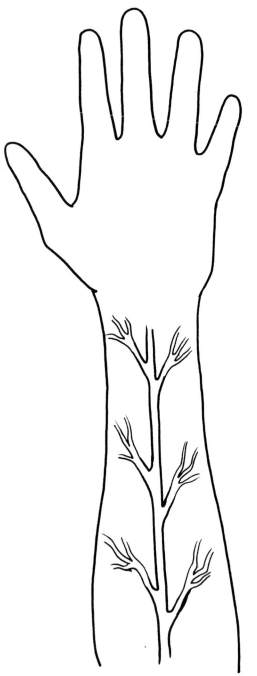

Fig. 2.87 The vasculature is unaffected by mild swelling in the forearm.

necrosis occurs in the flexor muscles, the median and ulnar nerve and in the most severe cases even the skin. Gangrene and amputation can follow. Necrotic muscle becomes replaced with extensive scarring with the wrist and fingers becoming contracted and insensitive (Fig. 2.85).

There are lesser forms of the condition in which only part of the flexors necrose and contract. There may be sparing of the median and ulnar nerves which are relatively less sensitive than muscle to loss of blood supply. Complete obstruction of the brachial artery will cause muscle necrosis within a few hours. Venous and capillary obstruction is probably tolerated for more than twenty four hours. Beware of the vicious circle of oedema – compression – ischaemia–more oedema etc. This is identical in all 'compartment syndromes'.

TREATMENT

1. **Prevention. There has not been a case of Volkmann's contracture in the past twenty years since we brought in the following rules in our emergency department:**
   a. **No recent fracture has a full plaster applied, only slabs or fully split and opened casts.**
   b. **All limbs are padded before the application of casts.**
   c. **All limbs are elevated for twelve hours and a circulation check is carried out in hospital or at home for more simple fractures. Active movement of fingers and toes is encouraged.**
   d. **All outpatients are checked within twelve to eighteen hours, but have written instructions to return if there are signs of vascular problems (increased pain, swelling, blue-**

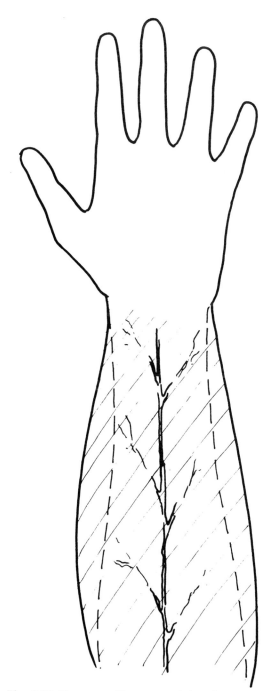

Fig. 2.88 Gross swelling or a tight plaster or a tight fascial compartment cause the smaller vessels to be compressed and circulation in these vessels ceases.

ness or excess pallor, numbness, or loss of capillary return).

2. If in doubt explore the artery. Explore early rather than procrastinate. However in the case of a supracondylar fracture of the humerus:
   a. Undo the flexed elbow and remove all plaster and bandages.
   b. Elevate the hand and get the child actively moving the fingers if possible.
   c. If the circulation improves then put the child in overhead traction with an ulna screw (Fig. 2.82).
   d. If there is no improvement explore the artery as outlined in acute vascular problems.
   e. In delayed cases, or if the circulation does not return fully and freely, split the fascia in the forearm very widely both anteriorly and posteriorly (Fig. 2.89). Surgical exploration should extend to the flexor

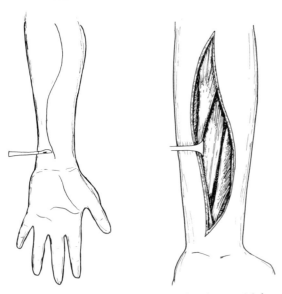

Fig. 2.89 The incision for fascial release. Make sure the decompression is thorough and goes down to the deepest muscles.

digitorum profundus and to the flexor pollicus longus which sustain the maximum damage. Leave the wounds open until the swelling subsides, then secondarily close the wounds or apply skin grafts.

(iii) Established Volkmann's contracture

This condition comes in many degrees of severity. In the lesser forms where there is a viable limb with some sensation, the function can be improved by excision of the contracted muscle groups. This will have three effects:

1. It will allow better excursion of the fingers.
2. It will allow the use of undamaged muscle.
3. The median nerve which is often caught up in the scar tissue can be freed and sensation may improve.

KEY POINTS

a. The flexor digitorum profundus and the flexor pollicus longus are most often affected and may need to be excised.
b. In more severe cases the superficialis and even some of the extensors may be scarred and non-contractile.
c. As long as there is protective sensation excise the dead and contracted muscle and rearrange what is left of functioning muscles to at least give some active flexion and extension of the fingers.
d. A muscle slide detaching the flexor muscles from their origin on the medial epicondyle and the interosseous membrane will allow greater finger movement (Fig. 2.90).

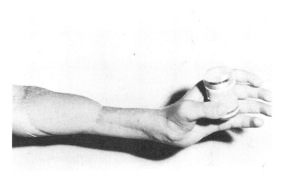

Fig. 2.90 This severe Volkman's contracture has undergone excision of dead and contracted muscle and a muscle slide.

(iv) Difficulties in reduction

This is a fracture that can usually be reduced into anatomical position with care and skill. The techniques are basically those of traction, reduction of the lateral or medial shift and then direct pressure on the olecranon pushing the distal fragment anteriorly whilst flexing the elbow (Fig. 2.91 (a),(b) and (c)).

Problems encountered include the very fat arm, or the very grossly swollen arm which will almost require extrasensory perception to give you the feel that the fracture has been reduced. Remember that it is better to put the fat arm or the grossly swollen arm in overhead traction rather than accept poor position that is likely to deteriorate as the swelling goes down.

(v) Redisplacement

Fractures that are well reduced and are able to be flexed at the elbow and maintained in reasonable flexion generally will not slip. Fractures that tend to slip are those with only partial reduction and especially those with any persistent rotary displacement. Remember the distal end of the humerus is very narrow in cross section in the supracondylar region (Fig. 2.92). All parents should be warned of the possibility that the fracture may slip and that a further reduction may be necessary. The important point is not that

TREATMENT

All supracondylar fractures have to be maintained in good position in both the anteroposterior and lateral views. Pay particular attention to see that rotation is normal. Radiographs should be done at the time of reduction and three days later. Reduce the fracture a second time if necessary. Internal fixation is not necessarily indicated if a fracture redisplaces, however satisfactory reduction must be achieved the second time around. Any instability at that stage does call for fixation by crossed Kirschner wires.

you have to reduce the fracture again but that the final reduction of the fracture is correct.

(vi) Malunion

If malunion occurs in a supracondylar fracture it is because reduction of the fracture and maintenance of the position is not satisfactory.

Cubitus varus (Fig. 2.93) produces an ugly arm known as a gunstock deformity and is due to accepting a gap on the lateral side at the fracture site often with some rotation (Fig. 2.94).

This deformity occurs in those fractures in which the original displacement of the distal fragment is posterior and medial.

It is important to use the posterior and medial periosteal hinge (Fig. 2.95). The lateral gap is closed by holding the elbow both in flexion and with the forearm in full pronation (that is with the hand facing away from the body) (Fig. 2.96).

Cubitus valgus is due to accepting a gap on the medial side of the fracture site allowing an increased carrying angle at the elbow. Minor degrees of this deformity (Fig. 2.97) are much more acceptable than the gunstock (varus) deformity.

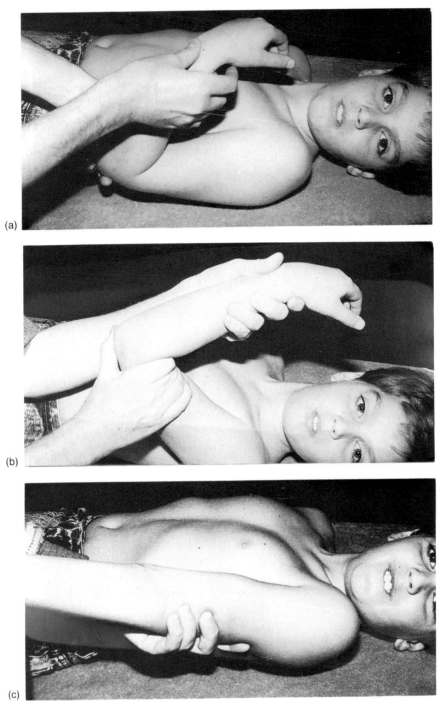

Fig. 2.91 This series shows the steps in reduction of a supracondylar fracture of the humerus: (a) alignment of the humerus; (b) direct pressure over the olecranon while traction is maintained; (c) flexion to a safe point as far as circulation will allow.

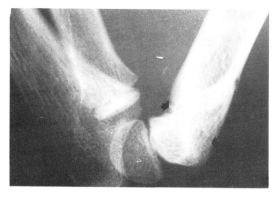

Fig. 2.92 The maintenance of position in a supracondylar fracture is difficult due to the small surface area of the distal humerus.

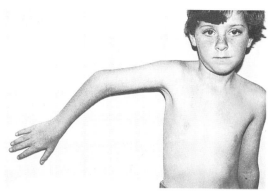

Fig. 2.93 Cubitus varus or gunstock deformity after malunion of a supracondylar fracture.

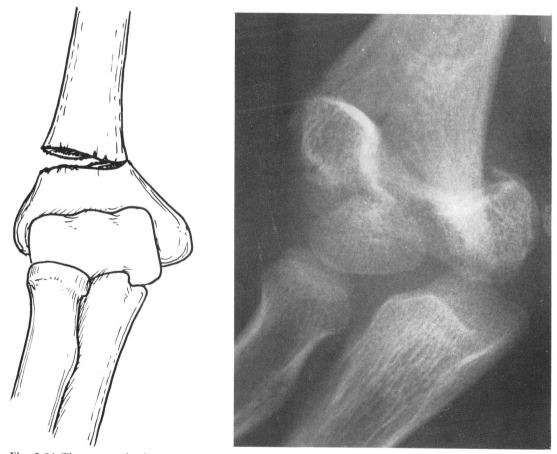

Fig. 2.94 The cause of cubitus varus. Accepting poor position of the fracture by leaving a gap laterally.

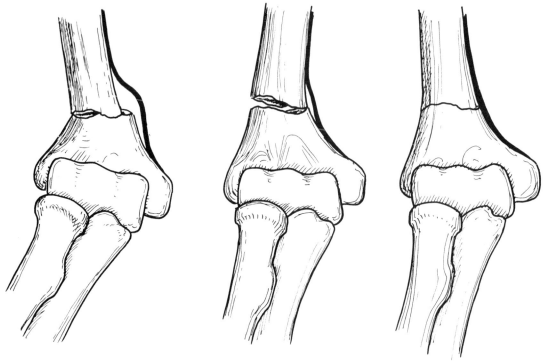

Fig. 2.95 The use of the periosteal hinge in reduction of supracondylar fractures.

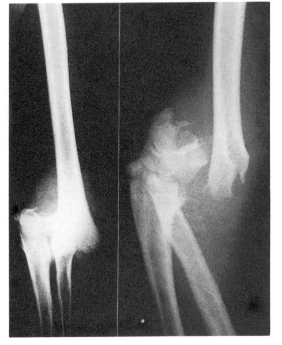

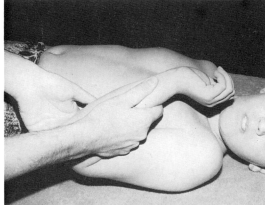

Fig. 2.96 The position of immobilization of a supracondylar fracture of the humerus (medial and posterior displacement) after reduction. Note that the palm faces away from the patient thus closing the gap on the lateral side and tightening the medial periosteal hinge.

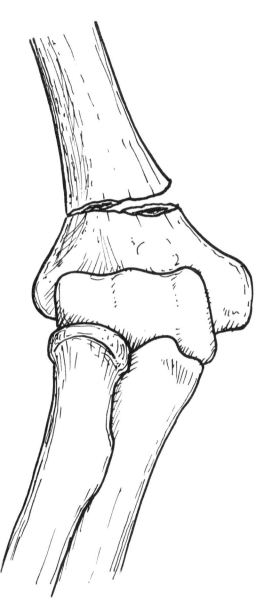

Fig. 2.97 The gap is on the opposite side to the periosteal hinge. Lateral displacement means lateral hinge.

Cubitus valgus occurs when the fracture is displaced posteriorly and laterally (Fig. 2.98) and a gap is left on the medial side after reduction. In this case the hinge is posterior and lateral. The gap is held closed by fully supinating the forearm and immobilizing the elbow flexed and with the hand facing the patient (Fig. 2.99).

Rotation of the distal fragment is difficult to judge on the anteroposterior view, however it is clearly seen on the lateral radiograph of the elbow (Fig. 2.100).

TREATMENT OF MALUNION _____

Corrective osteotomy is indicated for cosmetic reasons in cubitus varus and the more severe degrees of cubitus valgus and other deformities.

KEY POINTS

a. **Correction is best done just above the supracondylar area.**
b. **A closing wedge osteotomy leaving an intact periosteum on the opposite cortex is best.**
c. **Insert a screw in the distal fragment at 90° to the bone surface prior to the osteotomy.**
d. **Outline the wedge to be removed with multiple drill holes and remove the wedge using a sharp osteotome.**
e. **Insert a screw in the proximal fragment and wire the two screws together. This uses the intact periosteum on the opposite cortex to help stabilize the osteotomy (Fig. 2.101).**
f. **Rotation and extension deformity can be corrected by shaping the wedge.**
g. **Fixation of the osteotomy can also be done with staples, lag screws or Kirschner wires.**

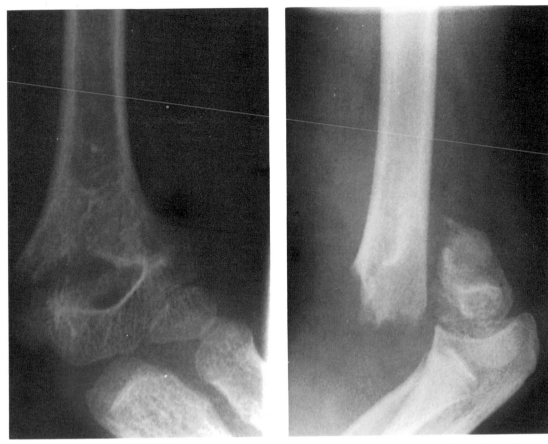

Fig. 2.98 The type of supracondylar fracture that is likely to lead to cubitus valgus (posterior and lateral displacement).

(vii) Nerve injuries

In my experience the median nerve is the most frequently injured nerve associated with this fracture, although other authors quote the radial nerve as being more frequently involved.

The median nerve is separated from the sharp anterior edge of the proximal fragment by a thin sheet of the brachialis muscle and along with the brachial artery is very vulnerable to stretching and even being impaled on the proximal fragment.

TREATMENT

Almost all nerve lesions associated with this fracture are in the form of neuropraxia rather than actual division of the nerve. Recovery can be anticipated in six weeks or less. If the lesion fails to improve in that time electromyographic studies should be done and if they confirm a block, exploration of the nerve is advised.

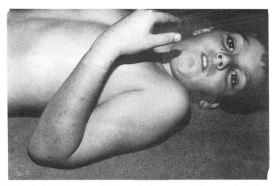

Fig. 2.99 The position of the arm after reduction of a supracondylar fracture with posterior and medial displacement. The palm faces towards the patient.

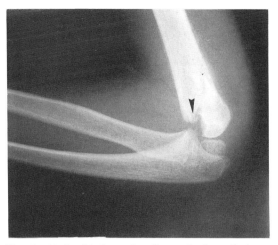

Fig. 2.100 In this lateral radiograph there is some rotation of the distal fragment.

(viii) Myositis ossificans

A small amount of ectopic bone is not infrequent after this fracture, but severe calcification and ossification in the brachialis is rare. It can follow repeated and rough manipulation of the fracture.

TREATMENT

This is only indicated when the bone acts as a block to flexion and is discrete. It should then be excised.

> ## KEY POINTS
> a. **Let the bone mature for twelve to eighteen months.**
> b. **Excise the bone cleanly and obtain careful haemostasis.**
> c. **Start early mobilization of the elbow.**

(ix) Stiffness of the elbow

This is an intra-articular fracture so that some stiffness is to be expected. Indeed given the displacement of some fractures it is surprising to see the excellent range of movement that is usually obtained (Figs 2.102 and 2.103).

TREATMENT

Stiffness after the fracture has united will respond to active movements if the problem is scarring in the soft tissues. Passive stretching is banned as it simply increases the stiffness by tearing the soft tissues instead of stretching them.

Most children will regain all possible movement within twelve months if they actively exercise the elbow. If loss of movement persists beyond this time it is seldom more than 20–30° of extension and 10° of flexion.

A single passive stretching of the elbow under anaesthesia after twelve months has passed is worthwhile. Follow this up with active exercises.

Occasionally loss of flexion is due to posterior angulation at the fracture site (Fig.2.104). Rarely an osteotomy is indicated.

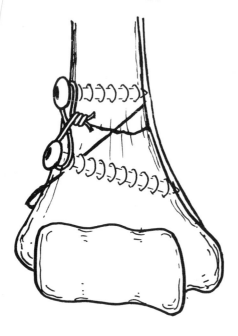

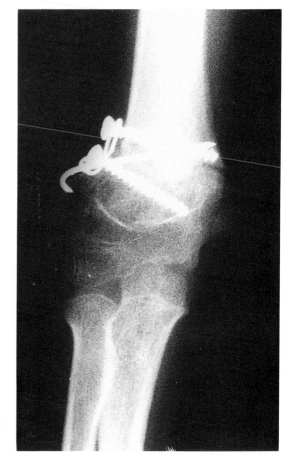

Fig. 2.101 Simple method of fixation after a corrective osteotomy. The medial cortex should have a greenstick fracture and intact periosteum.

2.3.2 CONDYLAR AND SUPRACONDYLAR IN ADULTS

Malunion

Comminuted fractures of the lower end of the humerus (Fig. 2.105) are intra-articular and therefore require accurate reduction and fixation if malunion is to be avoided.

Once malunion has occurred there is little that can be done and poor function is inevitable.

2.3.3 SHAFT

Complications occur frequently with these fractures, and include:

1. Delayed and non union
2. Malunion
3. Nerve injuries
4. Vascular injuries
5. Pathological fractures

(i) Delayed and non union

This problem occurs quite frequently in fractures of the humerus and is mainly associated with the difficulties of immobilization of this bone.

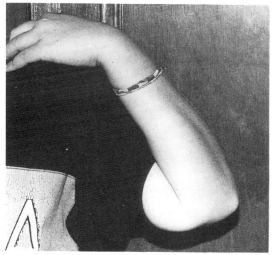

Fig. 2.102 Normal range of flexion of the elbow after a supracondylar fracture.

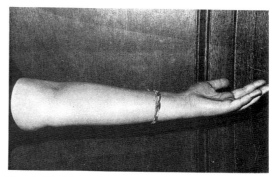

Fig. 2.103 Normal range of extension (some months) after a supracondylar fracture.

TREATMENT

As for all delayed and non union the treatment is by open reduction, internal fixation and bone grafting.

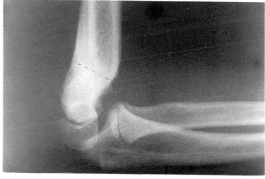

Fig. 2.104 This fracture has posterior angulation and this will result in hyperextension and loss of flexion of the elbow.

KEY POINTS

a. **The humerus is a difficult bone to internally fix due to its shape, and difficulty in access particularly in relation to the radial nerve (Fig. 2.106).**

b. **Access to fractures of the distal end of the humerus is either through a triceps splitting incision or by taking off the olecranon by osteotomy (with a predrilled screw hole in place for the repair) and turning back the whole of the triceps. This gives access to the complete articular surface of the distal end of the humerus (Figs 2.107 and 2.108 (a) and (b).**

c. **Access to the shaft of the humerus.**
   i. **In the distal half safe access is best through a posterior incision which splits the triceps. The proximal end of this incision endangers the radial nerve. The radial nerve must be identified and protected in the groove on the humeral shaft. Often the fracture makes it hard to pick up the nerve at this point so that it is usually easier to identify the radial**

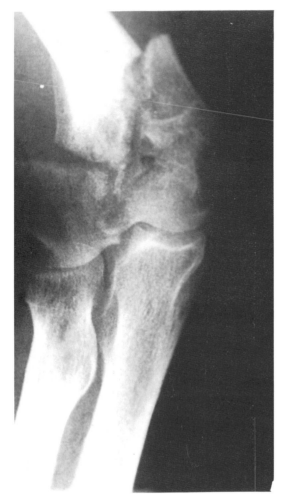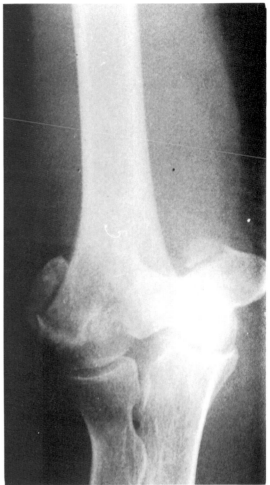

Fig. 2.105 Some of the many types of comminuted fractures of the distal third of the humerus. The restoration of the articular surface is important.

nerve as it pierces the lateral intermuscular septum and trace it back to the fracture site.

ii. In the more proximal fractures an anterior incision starting in the delto-pectoral groove can be extended both proximally (turning back the clavicular origin of the deltoid) and distally towards the deltoid insertion and along the outer border of the biceps (Fig. 2.106).

(ii) Malunion

The humerus can unite with lateral, medial anterior or posterior angulation or a rotary deformity. There can also be combinations of the above. Shortening is not a problem and is not readily detectable.

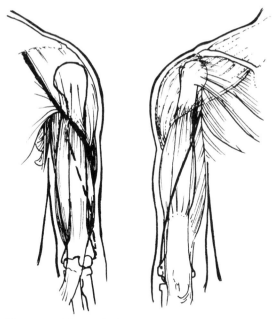

Fig. 2.106 The radial nerve and its relationship to the humerus is shown both from anterior and posterior aspects. The proximal heavy line is the skin incision for access to the proximal end of the humerus.

TREATMENT

1. **Prevention of angulation and rotary deformity is important and is not difficult. If the fracture is so unstable that the deformity cannot be held in plaster, then open reduction and internal fixation is indicated.**
2. **Deformity, if noticeable, must be corrected either by osteoclasis and plaster immobilization or by osteotomy at the fracture site, correction and internal fixation.**

(iii) Nerve lesions

Approximately 5% of fractures of the humerus result in damage to the radial nerve. In most cases the lesion is either a stretching or a bruising of the nerve with temporary loss of

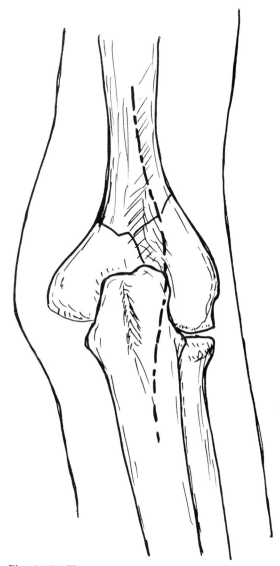

Fig. 2.107 The incision for access to the distal half of the humerus.

function and rapid and spontaneous recovery.

The diagnosis is obvious as high radial nerve lesions have wrist drop due to the temporary (or permanent) loss of nerve supply to the extensors of the wrist and metacarpophalangeal joints of the fingers. A small area of sensation is lost on the dorsal aspect over the base of the thumb (Fig. 2.109).

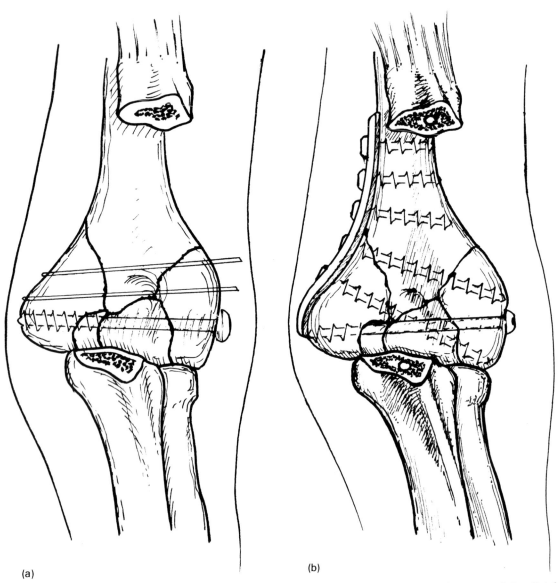

(a)   (b)

Fig. 2.108 (a) the method of reduction; (b) the method of fixation of comminuted fractures of the distal humerus. Note the olecranon has been osteotomized after being predrilled for easy reduction and fixation.

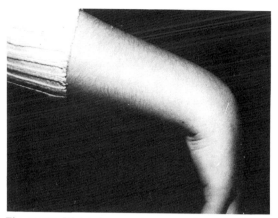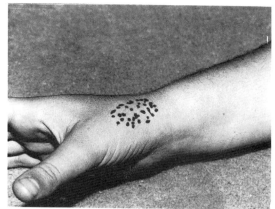

Fig. 2.109 Wrist drop and sensory loss are the signs of a radial nerve lesion.

TREATMENT

Since most lesions spontaneously recover within six weeks all that is necessary is to prevent contraction of unopposed muscles. I prefer to do this by having the patient continuously passively extend the wrist and fingers or to use a lively splint. Such a splint allows active flexion of the wrist and has elastic or springs to take the place of the extensors. The alternative use of a cock-up splint holds the wrist and fingers passively extended but does not allow activity.
   Signs of recovery.

a. Sensory loss over the base of the thumb tends to fade and disappear.

b. A flicker of power in the wrist extensors usually occurs two to three weeks after the sensory loss starts to improve.

c. Electromyography will show the earliest signs of recovery and should be repeated at six weekly intervals in cases where clinical signs of recovery are delayed.

The indications for exploration of the radial nerve are clearcut.

1. Compound fractures even where the radial nerve is not involved, it is important to visualize the nerve to see that it is not involved in the wound or the fracture. The decision to explore the radial nerve is absolute in those cases of compound fractures of the shaft of the humerus that have clinical evidence of nerve damage (e.g. wrist drop).

2. All open reductions of fractures of the shaft of the humerus must be planned to avoid damage to the radial nerve (see below). The only way you can be sure of avoiding the nerve in most cases is to find the nerve and protect it.

3. In closed fractures with radial nerve lesions the nerve will need to be explored only occasionally. The indications here are failure of the nerve to recover after 12 weeks, with no evidence of recovery on the E.m.g. Longitudinal fractures are more likely to have physical damage to the nerve than transverse fractures.

KEY POINTS

a. **The radial nerve curls around the humerus being closely applied to the posterior and lateral aspects of the middle third of the bone (Fig. 2.106).**

b. **A short spiral fracture (Fig. 2.110) with displacement can stretch or even cut the radial nerve. It can get caught up in the callus at the fracture site and need to be dissected out carefully. Where the nerve is cut repair is essential using microsurgical techniques. If there is a problem getting end to end anastamosis without tension then the nerve can be transposed through the fracture site or around the humerus to give extra length and allow resection of any neuroma.**

(iv) Brachial plexus and vascular lesions

Brachial plexus traction injuries occur occasionally in fractures of the humerus. These injuries have a poor prognosis.

In compound fractures with wounds on the medial or anterior aspects of the humerus, nerve and brachial artery injury are not uncommon (Fig. 2.111).

TREATMENT _____

As with all compound fractures the wound must be carefully explored and all damaged structures repaired.

(v) Pathological fractures

Metastatic lesions in the humerus which predispose to fractures are commonly from breast and lung carcinoma.

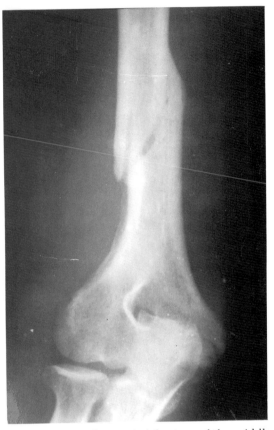

Fig. 2.110 The short spiral fracture of the middle third of the humerus is commonly associated with radial nerve lesions.

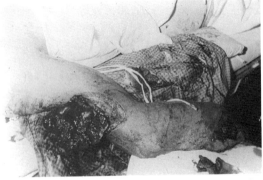

Fig. 2.111 Brachial artery injury associated with a severe compound fracture of the humerus.

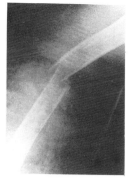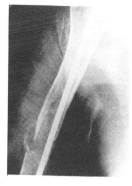

Fig. 2.112 Internal fixation with the use of acrylic cement to fill a defect due to a metastasis and provide stability and mobility for a patient with a limited life span.

TREATMENT

Aggressive treatment of pathological fractures of the humerus is indicated where the general condition of the patient is satisfactory. Open reduction, internal fixation (sometimes with the use of filling material such as bone cement or ceramic spacers) and local anti-tumour therapy form the basis of treatment (Fig. 2.112).

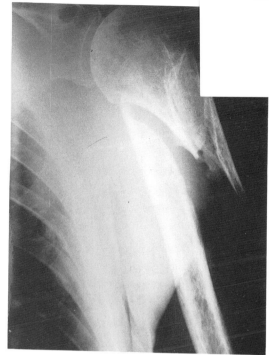

Fig. 2.113 Widely displaced fractures below the neck of the humerus commonly have soft tissue interposition.

2.3.4 FRACTURES OF THE NECK AND HEAD OF THE HUMERUS

The following are the major complications:

1. Non union and malunion
2. Pain and stiffness
3. Damage to the axillary nerve
4. Vascular and brachial plexus damage
5. Avascular necrosis

(i) Non union and malunion

Non union is seen occasionally in these fractures and may be due to soft tissue interposition of the long head of the biceps tendon or a piece of deltoid muscle (Fig. 2.113).

TREATMENT

Non union may be painless and a moderate range of movement may persist at the false joint. Usually it is painful and requires open reduction and internal fixation.

KEY POINTS

a. **Use an incision in the deltopectoral groove and elevate the clavicular origin of the deltoid to allow greater visibility (Fig. 2.106).**

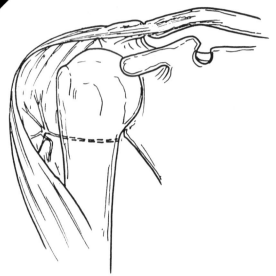

Fig. 2.114 Note the position of the axillary nerve as it passes through the quadrilateral space on the medial and posterior aspects of the neck of the humerus and supplies the deltoid.

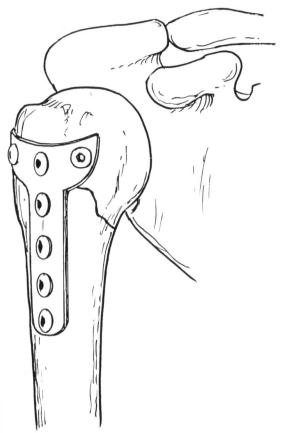

Fig. 2.115 Many displaced fractures of the neck of the humerus in younger fit patients should have open reduction and plating.

b. **Carefully reduce the fracture taking care not to damage the nerve supply to the deltoid (the axillary nerve which is close to the neck of the humerus) (Fig. 2.114).**

c. **Fixation of the fracture requires skill and sometimes ingenuity. If the bone is strong enough use a T shaped buttress plate and splay the cancellous screws in the head of the humerus (Fig. 2.115).**

Malunion of fractures of the head and neck of the humerus is often present to a limited degree, as the fractures are seldom reduced anatomically. The head of the humerus is so well covered by articular cartilage and the range of movement is normally so great that some malunion can exist without affecting the function of the shoulder to a great degree. We are also dealing with an age group (over 60) with these fractures that accept some loss of function without having to alter their life-style.

If the bone is soft or comminuted then wire loop tension bands or combined wire loop and screw or rod fixation may be necessary. As the bone is cancellous, grafting is not necessary unless there is a gap (Fig. 2.116).

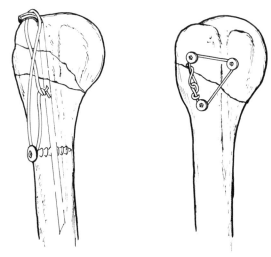

Fig. 2.116 Some other methods of fixation of the head of the humerus such as wires and screws and Rush nails may be necessary.

TREATMENT

Malunion of comminuted fractures such as the four part fracture (Fig. 2.117) may require operative treatment due to severe and disabling pain associated with joint incongruity. The choice of operations lies between arthrodesis and a resurfacing prosthesis.

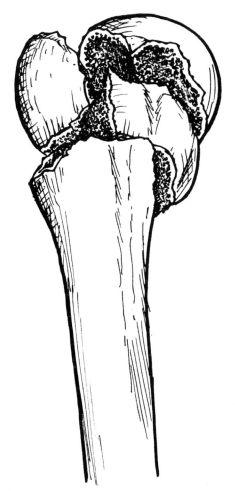

Fig. 2.117 The worst fracture of the humeral head: the four part fracture.

KEY POINTS

a. **Arthrodesis of the shoulder is a major procedure which will relieve pain but only give very limited 'movement' of the shoulder (actually scapular rotation).**

b. **If an arthrodesis is to be done I prefer to carry out a compression arthrodesis taking great care to set the shoulder in 50° of abduction, 40° of internal rotation and 25° of flexion (Fig. 2.118).**

c. **Prosthetic replacement is often used in four part fractures primarily. If there is severe malunion then some reconstruction of the proximal humerus using a bone graft may be necessary (Fig. 2.119). Replacement is also used in avascular necrosis of the humeral head.**

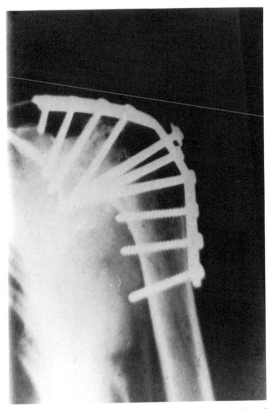

Fig. 2.118 Compression arthrodesis of the shoulder. Note that an anterior plate can be used as extra support if the bone is soft.

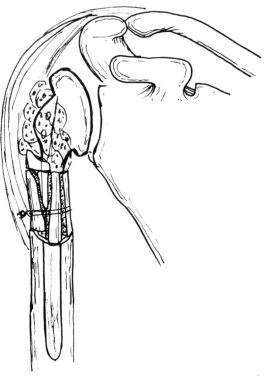

Fig. 2.119 Prosthetic replacement and bone grafting of the proximal humerus is used in some comminuted four part fractures and in tumour cases.

(ii) Pain and stiffness

This is the most common complication of fractures of the head and neck of the humerus. One reason can be a failure to reduce the component parts in a comminuted fracture giving a bony block. Mostly the stiffness that follows this fracture is due to adhesions within the joint and in the subacromial bursa. Pain can accompany this stiffness but mostly the stiffness and loss of function is not painful. Pain usually indicates either painful subacromial bursitis and adhesions or damage to the articular surface with the development of a traumatic arthritis.

TREATMENT

This is largely prophylactic:

1. **Reduce the fracture carefully.**
2. **If reduction is not possible by closed means then carry out open reduction if the patient is fit enough.**
3. **At least 75% of these fractures are undisplaced or minimally displaced, and as the fracture occurs through an area of bone that is largely cancellous, union will proceed rapidly. As soon as possible**

exercises to mobilize the shoulder should commence. The elbow, hand and fingers should be kept mobile with active exercises from day one.

4. Ten days after the fracture the arm should be put through pendulum exercises allowing swinging of the shoulder. This should progress with further active exercises and gentle stretching. Exercises should be carried out by the patient at home after a hot shower and should continue for about six months.

5. Gentle manipulation of the shoulder under an anaesthetic can be of value if stiffness persists. Great care needs to be taken to avoid refracturing the humerus.

(iii) Damage to the axillary nerve

This usually occurs at the time of injury. It can also be iatrogenic and care needs to be taken during reduction, particularly if it is an open reduction. The effect of damage to this nerve is to paralyse the deltoid muscle and therefore active abduction of the shoulder. Fortunately most times the nerve is not avulsed or divided but rather bruised and stretched. Most cases recover in six to ten weeks at least part of the power of the deltoid.

TREATMENT

In a young patient exploration of the nerve and even microsurgical repair has been carried out but so far the results of this line of treatment are not brilliant.

Some patients can cope without an active deltoid muscle by learning trick movements, whilst others are grossly disabled. The options if disability is severe are:

1. **Transfer the insertion of the trapezius into the humerus under the deltoid.**
2. **Arthrodesis of the shoulder (see Fig. 2.118).**

(iv) Vascular and brachial plexus damage

Again these injuries are most likely to occur at the time of injury but can also occur at operation. Compound wounds of the axilla associated with fractures of the head and neck of the humerus are highly likely to have such damage.

TREATMENT

Vascular damage (Fig. 2.120) is of course a surgical emergency and appropriate repair or grafting must be done. Nerve damage will similarly need repair.

— KEY POINTS —

a. **In order to obtain access to the vessels and brachial plexus it may be necessary to remove a segment of the clavicle (Fig. 2.121). Apply a semitubular plate over the segment and adjacent bone and having drilled and tapped all the screw holes you can easily reconstitute the clavicle after the repair.**

b. **As with all vascular and nerve repair associated with fractures stabilize the fracture (usually first).**

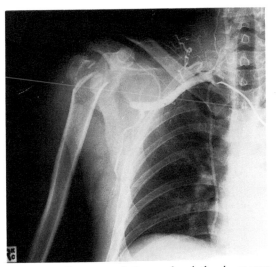

Fig. 2.120 Fracture of the neck of the humerus with damage to the axillary artery seen on an arteriogram (Dr J Harris' case).

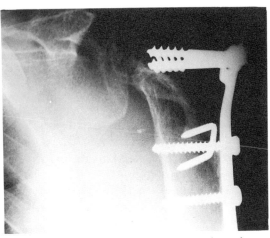

Fig. 2.122 The head of the humerus has almost completely disappeared in this patient who had a fracture dislocation treated by open reduction and fixation. There is a small irregular head and movement was limited and very painful. An arthroplasty was carried out.

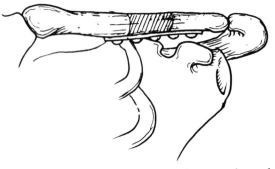

Fig. 2.121 To obtain access to the vessels and brachial plexus it may be necessary to remove a section of the clavicle. Drill and tap all screw holes prior to osteotomy of the clavicle and repair will be easy.

(v) Avascular necrosis

Avascular necrosis of the head or part of the head of the humerus can be a cause of pain and stiffness and of course incongruity of the articular surface (Fig. 2.122).

TREATMENT

Treatment of avascular necrosis is by either arthrodesis or arthroplasty (see above).

FURTHER READING

General

Charnley, J. (1970) *The Closed Treatment of Common Fractures*, 3rd edn, E. and S. Livingstone, Edinburgh.

Henry, A. K. (1979) *Extensile Exposures*, 2nd edn, Churchill Livingstone, Edinburgh.

Fingers, metacarpals and wrist

Heim, U. and Pfeiffer, K. M. (1988) *Internal Fixation of Small Fractures*, Springer-Verlag, Berlin.

Herbert, T. J. (1986) Use of the Herbert Bone Screw in Surgery of the Wrist, *Clin. Orthop.*, **202**, 79–92.

Children's fractures

Rang, M. (1986) *Children's Fractures*, 2nd edn, J. B. Lippincott, Philadelphia.

Rockwood, C. A., Wilkins, K. E. and King, R. E. (1984) *Fractures in Children*, J. B. Lippincott, Philadelphia.

Weber, B. G., Brunner, C. H. and Freuler, F. (1980) *Treatment of Fractures in Children and Adolescents*, Springer-Verlag, Berlin.

Adult's fractures

Brunner, Ch. F. and Weber, B. G. (1982) *Special Techniques in Internal Fixation*, Springer-Verlag, Berlin.

Edmonson, A. S. and Crenshaw, A. H. (1980) *Campbell's Operative Orthopaedics*, 6th edn, C. V. Mosby, St Louis.

CHAPTER THREE

Fractures of the trunk and spine

3.1 CLAVICLE

This is probably the most common fracture of childhood, and fortunately complications are rare.

Complications include:

1. Non union
2. Malunion
3. Nerve and vascular injuries

(i) Non union

This is almost unknown in children, but congenital pseudarthrosis of the clavicle can be mistaken for a non union (Fig. 3.1).

In adults non union can occur and is painful (Fig. 3.2).

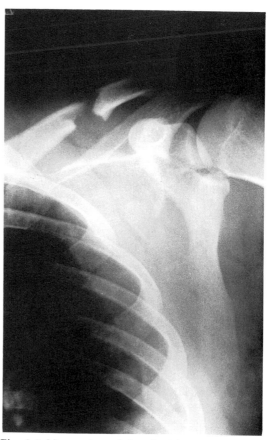

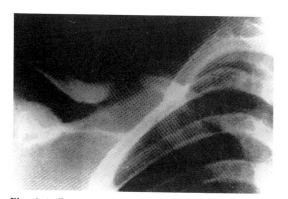

Fig. 3.1 Congenital pseudarthrosis of the clavicle.

Fig. 3.2 Non union of the clavicle in an adult.

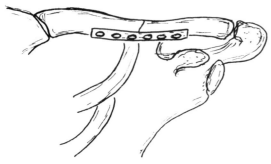

Fig. 3.3 Semi or one third tubular plate can be contoured to fit on the inferior surface of the clavicle.

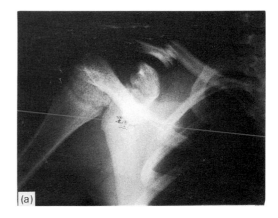

(a)

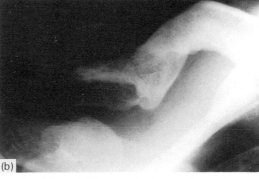

(b)

TREATMENT

Open reduction, plating and bone grafting will solve this problem.

> ## KEY POINTS
>
> a. **Use a skin incision above the clavicle. Try to avoid the supraclavicular nerves.**
> b. **The plate should be applied to the inferior aspect of the clavicle where possible and suitably contoured (Fig. 3.3). The bone graft material should be placed superiorly and posteriorly.**
> c. **Be aware of the neurovascular bundle that is inferior and posterior to the clavicle and protect these structures when drilling the screw holes.**

Fig. 3.4 (a) and (b) Shortening and overlap are common in clavicular fractures leading to malunion.

function and in some patients the cosmetic result does not seem to worry them. Given the choice of an operation and a scar or the bony prominence most elect to accept the deformity.

In young children there will be growth and moulding to smooth out the bump but in adults what you see at eight weeks is what you will have for the rest of the patient's life.

(ii) Malunion

Due to difficulties in immobilization many adult fractures of the clavicle unite with shortening, angulation and overlap (Fig. 3.4). In spite of this most patients will recover full

TREATMENT

Fractures of the clavicle that are overlapped or angulated are likely to leave a deformity that is unacceptable to (young) women. These frac-

tures have to be reduced and held in good position. If the fracture is treated with the arm in a sling in front of the body then some degree of malunion is inevitable.

In these circumstances uncomfortable as it is, some form of bracing the shoulders back is preferable (Fig. 3.5).

Once union is under way then it will be impossible to shift the fragments into alignment and the choice comes down to:

1. Open reduction and plating which will involve a scar and two operations (one to put the plate in and one to remove it 6−12 months later).
2. Allowing the fracture to unite as is and trimming the bony lump down to a smooth outline. This is the option that I generally adopt unless there is very gross deformity. You should wait for about 6 months after the fracture before carrying out this operation.

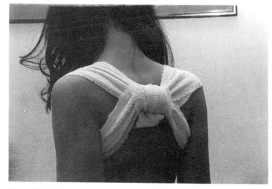

Fig. 3.5 Bracing a fractured clavicle with a figure of eight bandage. The axilla should be padded and the bandage should be of wide flannelette and not a soft crepe bandage as shown.

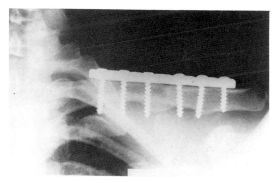

Fig. 3.6 This fractured clavicle has been trimmed and plated for better position. The plate would be better placed inferiorly.

KEY POINTS

a. Use a supraclavicular incision and try to avoid the supraclavicular nerves.
b. Always use an osteotome that is sharp and point it away from the subclavian vessels.
c. Trim the bone extensively. In some cases with gross overlap and anterior prominence (Fig. 3.6) an osteotomy and internal fixation will give a better cosmetic result.
d. Use a subcuticular suture in the skin.

(iii) Nerve and vascular injuries

Comminuted fractures in adults can be associated with nerve and vascular damage. Beware particularly of a sharp spike of bone pointing inferiorly (Fig. 3.7).

TREATMENT

Acute nerve and vascular damage will be noted at the time of admission to the emergency room and appropriate action taken. Vascular damage

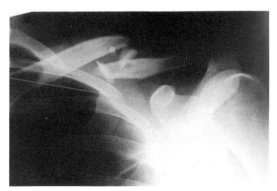

Fig. 3.7 Note the sharp spike of bone pointing towards the neurovascular structures which are inferior and posterior to the middle third of the clavicle.

must be repaired, whilst nerve damage will need to be assessed to see if it represents local damage to the brachial plexus with continuing compression by the fracture fragments or an associated avulsion injury of the nerve roots.

Occasionally in displaced fractures with a lot of callus a compression syndrome can develop as the brachial plexus and the subclavian vessels become squeezed between the callus and the first rib (or even a cervical rib and band). In these circumstances a decompression operation will be necessary.

3.2 SCAPULA

These fractures are uncommon and the complications are therefore rare. They include:

1. Non union.
2. Shoulder instability in glenoid fractures.

(i) Non union

Many fractures of the scapula unite by fibrous union and this in itself causes no problem in fractures of the body of the scapula. However fractures of the acromion and of the coracoid process (Fig. 3.8 (a) and (b)) will not unit if displaced and may be painful. In addition fractures of the glenoid (Fig. 3.9) will not unite if displaced and being intra-articular fractures may cause pain and instability (see below).

TREATMENT

All displaced fractures of the acromion, coracoid process and glenoid require open reduction and screw fixation initially. Non unions that are painful will require freshening of the fracture site and fixation with screws (Fig. 3.10).

(ii) Shoulder instability in glenoid fractures

Fractures of the glenoid rim are often associated with stripping and tearing of the labrum glenoidale and may result in instability of the shoulder joint.

TREATMENT

It is important to recognize this potential problem and to carry out open reduction primarily (Fig. 3.11).

Secondary reconstruction is difficult; it may be necessary to do an osteotomy of the neck of the scapula and bone graft.

3.3 SPINE

3.3.1 CERVICAL SPINE

There are some horrendous complications of spinal injuries. Most of the neurological problems arise at the time of injury, and I will not

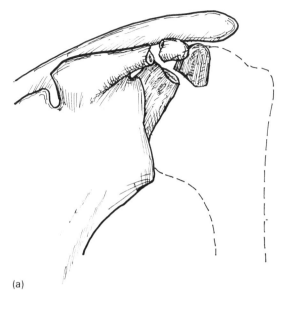

(a)

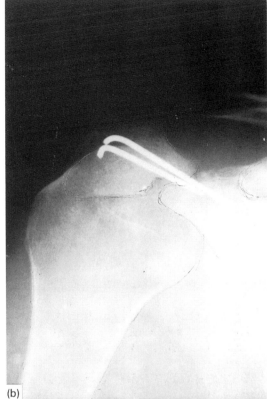

(b)

Fig. 3.8 (a) Displaced fractures of the coracoid process and the acromion; (b) note the acromion fracture has been pinned poorly as the fracture is held apart.

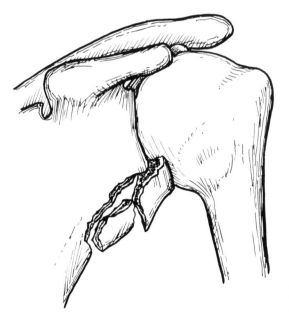

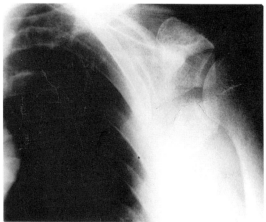

Fig. 3.9 Fractures of the scapula involving the glenoid.

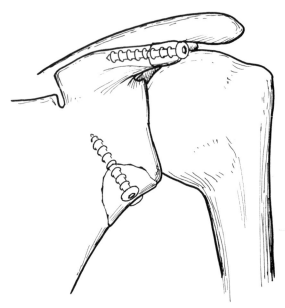

Fig. 3.10 Internal fixation after accurate reduction.

discuss the management of partial or complete paraplegia or quadriplegia with all their own complications. Such patients require the dedicated medical and nursing skills of a special spinal unit from the outset.

As with all spinal fractures and fracture dislocations the important decisions regarding treatment revolve around these questions:

1. Is the fracture/dislocation *stable*?
2. Is there a neurological deficit?

If there is a major neurological deficit then arrange transfer of the patient to a special unit. Immobilize the neck in a collar and arrange a medical escort to ensure careful handling of the patient so that the neurological deficit is not worsened.

The following fractures are stable:

1. Chip and crush fractures of the vertebral body without fractures of the posterior elements (Fig. 3.12).

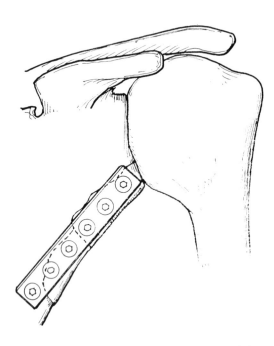

Fig. 3.11 Open reduction and fixation to stabilize the shoulder joint.

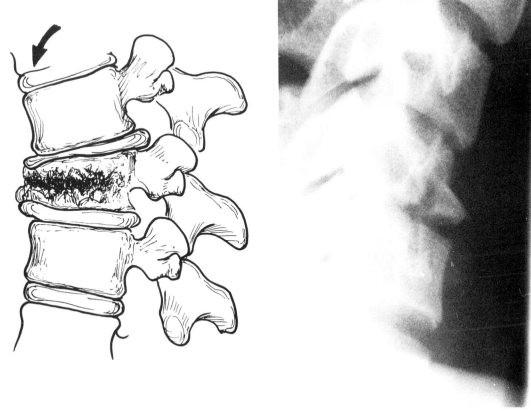

Fig. 3.12 Crush fractures of the cervical spine.

2. Isolated fractures of the appendages, such as spinous processes or transverse processes (Fig. 3.13).

Stable fractures without neurological symptoms or signs require immobilization only in a cervical collar (Fig. 3.14).

An unstable fracture is defined as one which by a change in its position has the potential to cause the development of or increase in neural deficit.

The following fractures and dislocations are *unstable*:

1. Fractures of the posterior elements (especially bilaterally) (Fig. 3.15).
2. Comminuted (teardrop) fractures of the vertebral body.

3. Crush fractures associated with fractures of the posterior elements (Fig. 3.16).
4. All dislocations (Fig. 3.17).
5. Fractures of the odontoid process (Fig. 3.18).

All unstable fractures and dislocations and fracture/dislocations without neurological problems require skull traction or halo traction initially. They may be maintained in traction until union and stability occurs, or may need a delayed spinal fusion.

Application of skull traction

Gardiner-Wells tongs are easily applied in the emergency room, requiring local anaesthesia

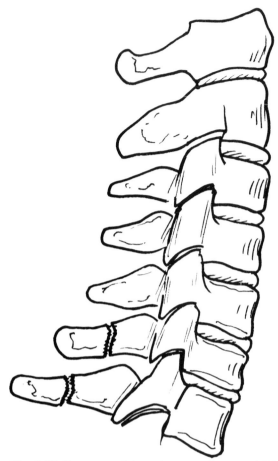

Fig. 3.13 Fractures of the spinous processes of C6 and C7 are common (clay shoveller's fractures).

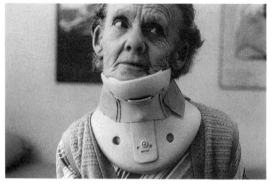

Fig. 3.14 Cervical collar to immobilize a stable neck fracture.

to be injected in the temporal ridge in line with the external auditory meatus and then the tightening of a knob on each side of the tongs. The instructions are on a plate welded to the tongs (Figs 3.19(a), (b) and (c)).

Complications of fractures and fracture/dislocations include:

1. Failure to reduce the fracture/dislocation.
2. Failure to maintain reduction.
3. Development of neurological symptoms and signs.
4. Pain and discomfort with activity after recovery.

(i) Failure to reduce a dislocation

This is usually due to locked facets. This can be unilateral or bilateral (Fig. 3.20). The general plan of reduction of a dislocation or fracture dislocation is to insert skull traction or a halo and apply traction of 8 kg. If the dislocation fails to reduce within six to eight hours then manual traction with some rotation under relaxant anaesthesia is usually successful.

TREATMENT

If traction is unsuccessful open reduction and unlocking of the facet is the next step.

─────────────────────

KEY POINTS

a. **The operation is carried out under general anaesthesia with the patient face down, using a midline posterior approach.**
b. **Extreme care needs to be taken in the moving and turning of the patient to avoid cord and nerve root damage.**
c. **If it is not easily determined the**

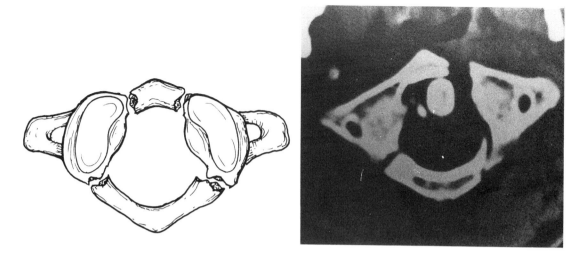

Fig. 3.15 CT scan of a bursting fracture of the atlas. This is an unstable fracture.

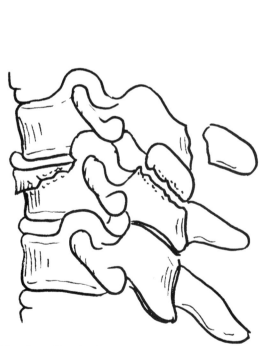

Fig. 3.16 Crush fracture with fracture of the posterior elements.

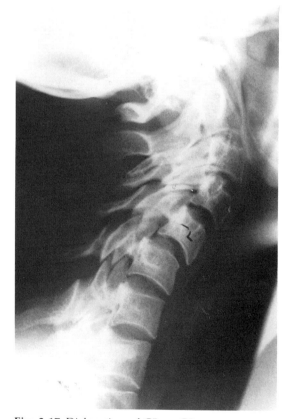

Fig. 3.17 Dislocation of C5 on C6.

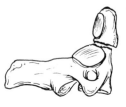

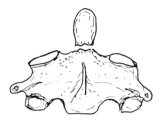

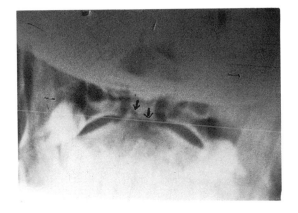

Fig. 3.18 Fracture of the odontoid process.

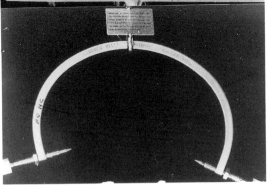

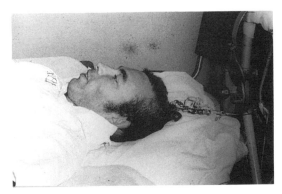

Fig. 3.19 Gardiner-Wells traction tongs for skull traction and their application.

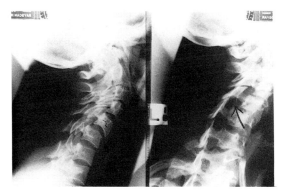

Fig. 3.20 Bilateral locked facets.

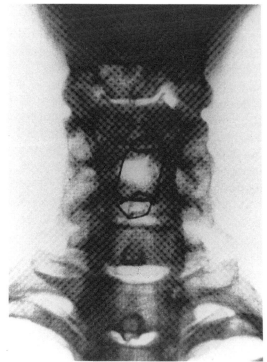

Fig. 3.21 Posterior wiring of spinous processes with bone grafting.

level can be checked on a mobile radiograph.

d. **Using a lever under the superior facet and traction the uni- or bilateral dislocations are easily reduced.**

e. **If you are unable to reduce easily then remove a small portion of the superior facet.**

f. **In bilateral cases and in fracture dislocations most surgeons now do a wiring of the spinous processes and a spinal fusion with graft material from the iliac crest (Fig. 3.21).**

(ii) Failure to maintain reduction

If closed reduction of a fracture dislocation or a dislocated cervical spine is successful then the subsequent maintenance of the position is important.

Failure is usually due to:

1. Taking the patient out of traction too soon. The initial traction must be maintained for ten to twelve weeks or until a jacket or a combined halo and jacket can be applied.

2. Taking the patient out of a jacket too soon. After reduction a body jacket holding the neck in some extension can be applied and must be maintained for 14–16 weeks to allow healing of the posterior ligaments. Spontaneous fusion anteriorly is a sign of stability. If it fails to occur then fusion should be carried out as a definitive procedure. Once the affected segment has fused then the patient can be advised to resume full activities including surfing and body contact sports.

3. Lack of immobilization after a primary fusion. Primary fusion and wiring needs six to eight weeks of immobilization in a collar to allow the graft to consolidate.

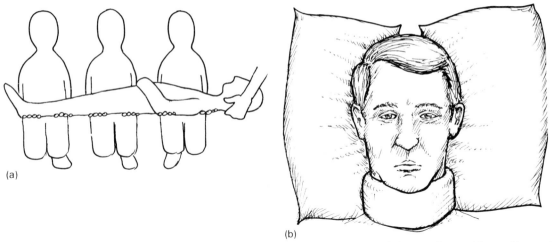

(a)

(b)

Fig. 3.22 (a) and (b) If possible immobilize neck injuries at the scene of the accident with a collar and pillows. To move the patient do not allow flexion or extension of the spine.

4. Early anterior fusion may increase instability by removing one of the only stable areas at that level. Early fusion should always be by posterior wiring and grafting.

(iii) Development of late neurological symptoms and signs

Neurological problems associated with fractures and dislocations of the cervical spine are usually those that occur at the time of injury. Our job is to protect the spinal cord and nerve roots at all times until full stability allows full activity.

Late neurological problems occur usually as a result of:

1. Failure to immobilize the injury at the scene of the accident and to transport the patient safely (Fig. 3.22(a) and(b)). If possible a collar should be applied at the scene of the accident to immobilize the neck. Extreme care should be taken to avoid flexing or extending the spine. The use of a Jordan frame (a metal frame that is placed around the patient whilst plastic struts which attach to the frame are slid under the patient) has simplified the transport of the injured patient.

2. In the hospital there can be failure to recognize a dislocation in the lower cervical spine and therefore failure to treat. Radiographs must show the whole cervical spine including C7 and T1 (Fig. 3.23). The doctor himself should supervise the patient in the radiography department to see that the spine is not flexed or extended until the radiographs show that there is no instability. Usually the lower cervical area can be vizualized by having the shoulders pulled down during the taking of the lateral films. CT scans can be of great assistance in deciding on the stability or otherwise of a fracture, and will also show if the spinal canal is compromised.

3. Failure to adhere to a proper treatment plan as discussed above.

All the above are preventable.

(iv) Pain and discomfort after recovery

At the completion of treatment in a fracture/dislocation or dislocation of the cervical spine

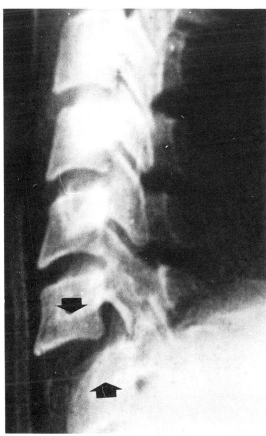

Fig. 3.23 The lateral view must go down to C7 otherwise the common C6 on C7 dislocation will be missed.

without neurological damage the patient should be pain free and able to carry out a normal social and working life.

In some patients managed conservatively where spontaneous fusion has not occurred, pain and discomfort develop as a result of either mild instability or due to damage and degeneration of the affected disc. Some patients develop nerve root irritation or compression.

TREATMENT _____

Spinal fusion of the affected segment will help these patients. In these late cases anterior spinal fusion with a dowel or block graft from the iliac crest is the best way to manage the problem (Fig. 3.24(a) and (b)).

3.3.2 THORACIC AND LUMBAR SPINES

Fractures in these areas of the spine are common, and fracture/dislocations are rare. Apart from paraplegia which will not be discussed, the major problem is, as in the cervical region, to decide if the lesion is stable or unstable.

Stable lesions:

1. Crush fractures of the body of a vertebra (flexion fractures) (Fig. 3.25).
2. Isolated fractures of the spinous and transverse processes (Fig. 3.26).

Unstable lesions (the potential for, or actual transverse displacement with possible cord and nerve root damage):

1. Compression (bursting) fractures, these often have cord damage due to displaced body fragments (Fig. 3.27).
2. All dislocations.
3. All fracture/dislocations
   Those associated with a lap seat belt may occur through soft tissue, or bone. It is a pure flexion injury over the seat belt and is known as a Chance fracture or fracture/dislocation (Fig. 3.28).
4. All fractures with involvement of both the vertebral body and the posterior elements (neural arch, associated processes and ligaments).
5. Some stable fractures which have been subjected to laminectomy become unstable because the posterior elements have now been compromised.

Complications of fractures and fracture/dislocations in the thoraco-lumbar region (apart from paraplegia which will not be discussed) include:

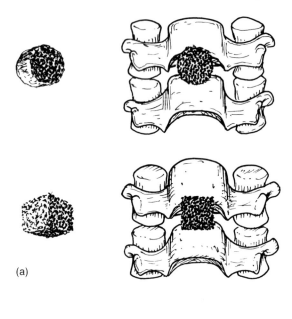

(a)

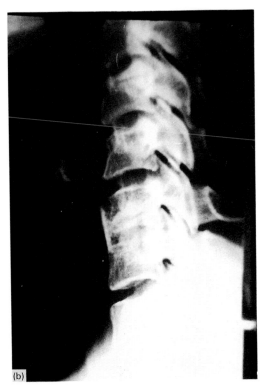

(b)

Fig. 3.24 (a) dowel or block grafts can be used for anterior spinal fusion; (b) anterior fusion of C5/6 and C6/7 using the dowel method of Cloward.

1. Stable lesions:
    (i) paralytic ileus
    (ii) thromboembolic problems
    (iii) severe angulation
    (iv) pathological fractures
    (v) residual back pain
2. Unstable lesions
    (vi) increased neurological deficit
    (vii) chronic instability (progressive deformity)

(i) Paralytic ileus

Paralytic ileus and gastric dilatation occur quite frequently in association with fractures in the thoraco-lumbar and lumbar regions due to retroperitoneal haemorrhage. The ileus is often short lived and can be managed by fluids only by mouth and observation. If gastric dilatation occurs then nasogastric suction and intravenous fluids may be required for three or four days.

(ii) Thromboembolic problems

Thromboembolic problems do occur in this group because they are kept in bed at rest for pain relief and in addition there can be localized thrombosis in the lumbar and pelvic region which can embolize. In some centres it is a routine for the patient to be on anticoagulants if there is a significant fracture in the thoraco-lumbar region. Anticoagulants should not be started for some 24 hours so as to avoid increasing local haemorrhage at the fracture site. In most centres elevation support of the lower limbs and early activity are used rather than anticoagulants.

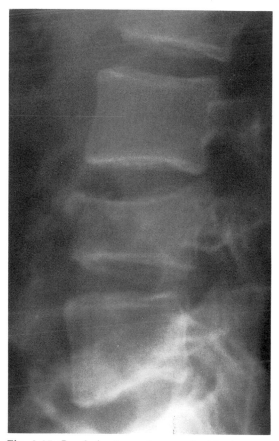

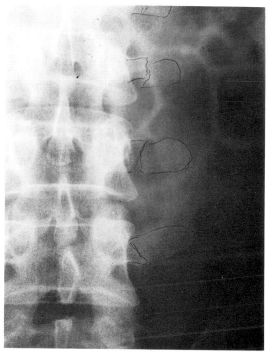

Fig. 3.26 Fractures of the transverse processes in the lumbar region indicate a severe soft tissue injury and is often associated with kidney damage.

Fig. 3.25 Crush fracture of a vertebral body.

(iii) Severe angulation

Although flexion type injuries are common (especially in the osteoporotic spine) most of these fractures initially involve a loss of anterior height of less than one third of the vertebral body. In the past there were attempts to try and restore the height of the vertebral body by such means as the use of plaster jackets applied on a table with the spine extended, or a Jewett hyperextension brace. The results were less than satisfactory as most of these patients needed to be kept in this immobilization for many months for it to be effective. The vertebral body tends to crush like a matchbox under your foot, and even though it can be pulled out it will collapse again in most cases once the immobilization has been removed. Currently most cases are treated with a period of rest followed by simple bracing for pain relief and then active exercises.

Under this regimen there may be some further loss of vertebral height and some angulation may occur. This is seldom a problem in non-pathological fractures but there have been cases of spinal cord compromise due to severe angulation (Fig. 3.29).

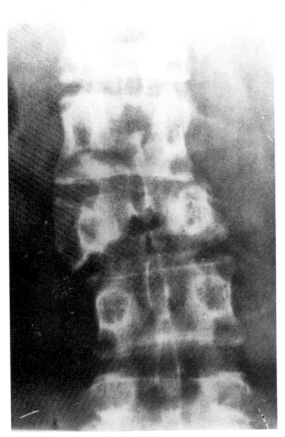

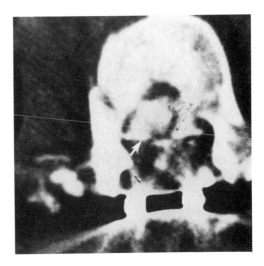

Fig. 3.27 Bursting fracture of T11. The CT scan shows displacement of a piece of the body with compromise of the spinal canal and cord.

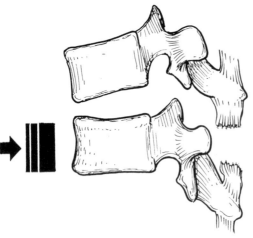

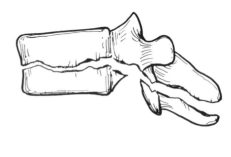

Fig. 3.28 The chance fracture.

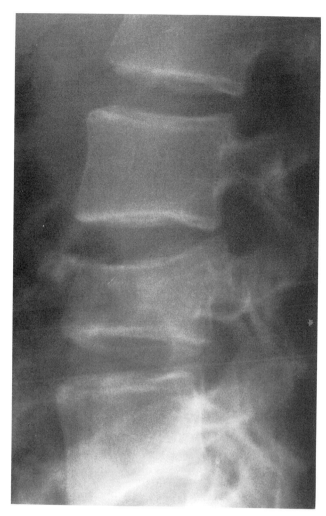

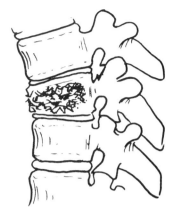

Fig. 3.29 Severe angulation of crushed vertebrae.

TREATMENT

Occasionally decompression of the spinal cord may be indicated together with a localized spinal fusion.

(iv) Pathological fractures

The thoracic and lumbar spines are commonly the site of pathological fractures. The commonest cause is post-menopausal osteoporosis. Other causes that are quite common include metastatic lesions from breast, prostate, lung and kidney malignancies (Fig. 3.30(a) and (b)). Multiple myeloma frequently presents as a pathological fracture in a porotic spine (Fig. 3.31).

The diagnosis of a pathological fracture must always be considered in the older age group. CT scans and nuclear scans are of great assistance in confirming a diagnosis (Fig. 3.32) of malignant disease although it can be hard to locate the primary tumour.

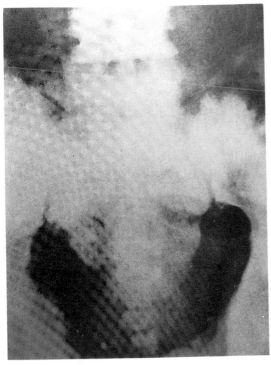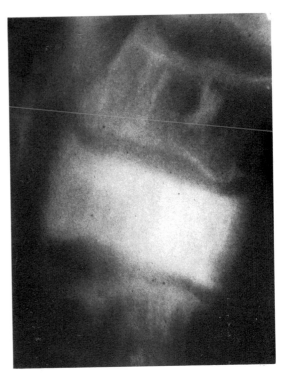

Fig. 3.30 Osteoblastic secondary deposits in the pelvis (a) and lumbar spines (b) from carcinoma of the prostate.

TREATMENT

Pathological fractures in osteoporosis have a good prognosis and require a short period of immobilization in a brace for pain relief, followed by a treatment for the osteoporosis. Currently we advise calcium, fluoride and a programme of active exercising, including if possible, swimming. Anabolic steroids and oestrogens have fallen out of favour.

Malignant lesions will require appropriate chemotherapy or radiotherapy locally plus whatever is appropriate for the primary tumour.

In most cases where the secondary lesion is in the bone the spinal cord is not threatened. Occasionally in addition to the bony lesion there is an invasive mass which causes spinal cord compression and requires decompression.

(v) Residual back pain

A common problem after a crush fracture or fractures of the transverse processes of the lumbar spines is an aching back after activity, prolonged standing or working in an awk-

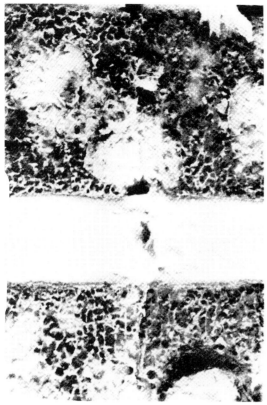

Fig. 3.31 Multiple myeloma in the lumbar spine.

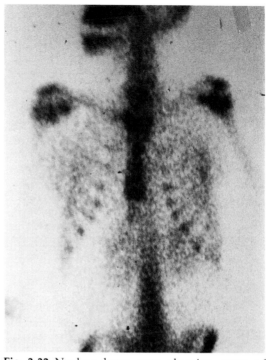

Fig. 3.32 Nuclear bone scan showing areas of increased uptake of the radioactive isotope in the lumbar spine and pelvis and other areas.

ward position. This can often be helped by strengthening the extensor muscles with physiotherapy and home exercises. Swimming is also of value as it seems to build up the extensor muscles with a non-violent exercise against the resistance of the water. It needs to be carried out for half an hour at least twice a week. Some patients find a lumbo-sacral support of value.

(vi) Increased neurological signs

Our goal in the management of all spinal injuries is to protect the spinal cord and nerve roots against further injury. The damage that has occurred in the original injury is unfortunate, any further deterioration in the neuro-

logical status is disastrous and basically preventable.

Problems can occur for the following reasons:

1. Failure to transport the patient properly from the scene of accident (see section on cervical spine).
2. Failure to recognize the nature of the lesion. This simply should not occur with the availability of radiographs and CT scans. The one circumstance that causes concern is the back injury patient that has a history of injury, a great deal of local pain, and apparently normal radiographs. This in fact can be an unstable fracture dislocation which is reduced when the

patient is lying flat. If there is severe pain take further radiographs including oblique films and CT scans to satisfy yourself that the spine is intact.

3. One rare but incontrovertible indication for decompression of the spinal cord is increasing neurological deficit. Laminectomy may however increase the instability.

(vii) Chronic instability

In unstable lesions in which fusion fails to develop there can be progressive deformity. Pain may increase and the cosmetic result can be unsatisfactory. Eventually if the deformity is sufficiently severe neurological deficit appears.

TREATMENT

Stabilization of the spine at an early stage is recommended. If the deformity has progressed to the stage of neurological deficit then recovery of the deficit is unlikely.

3.3.3 SACRUM AND COCCYX

A heavy fall onto the buttocks or a brutal kick can cause a fracture of the sacrum, or if lower down the coccyx. Sacral fractures can also be associated with severe crushing injuries of the pelvic ring.

Local pain is a feature of these fractures and the patient needs an inflatable ring on (and in) which to sit. Problems:

(i) Persistent pain
(ii) Local tenderness of the coccyx
(iii) Nerve root damage

(i) Persistent pain

Pain will often persist for years after an injury to the sacrum or coccyx. It is mostly related to sitting and to activity.

TREATMENT

Symptomatic treatment with analgesics and local heat has some value. Patients can be reassured that over a long period of time the symptoms do tend to ease.

(ii) Local tenderness of the coccyx

Local tenderness of the coccyx and coccydynia frequently follow displaced fractures of the coccyx. Sitting on a hard seat and having a bowel action can be extremely painful.

TREATMENT

Persistent local tenderness with anteversion of the fracture can make life miserable for your patient and justify excision of the distal fractured pieces of the coccyx.

KEY POINTS

a. **Place the patient in the lateral position with the buttocks strapped apart.**
b. **Use a longitudinal incision and dissect out the distal fragment using coagulation diathermy cautiously. Stay close to the bone as the rectum is a deep anterior relation of the coccyx.**
c. **Insert multiple deep sutures before tying them. (Not too deep as the rectum is not to far away.) This should completely eliminate the dead space and as there should be no bleeding, no drain is necessary.**

(iii) Nerve root damage

Damage to the first and second sacral nerve roots is a rare complication that produces sensory loss over the outer border of the foot some weakness of the hamstrings and gluteii, gross weakness of the calf muscles and loss of the ankle jerk.

TREATMENT

This is restricted to exercises.

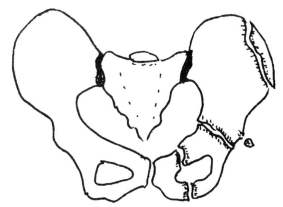

Fig. 3.33 Some of the many isolated fractures of the pelvis.

3.3.4 PELVIS

These fractures are common and mostly heal without complications, however there are many very serious complications that can occur. Often these fractures are not isolated injuries but are part of multi system trauma.

The complications include:

(i) Severe haemorrhage and shock
(ii) Thrombosis, and thromboembolism
(iii) Damage to pelvic organs and pelvic nerves
(iv) Damage to the bladder and urethra
(v) Infection in compound fractures
(vi) Malunion
(vii) Delayed union and non union
(viii) Damage to the hip joint

There are basically two types of fracture of the pelvis:

(a) Isolated fractures (Fig. 3.33).
(b) Fractures which disrupt the pelvic ring. These carry most of the complications (Fig. 3.34 (a),(b),(c),(d) and (e)).

(i) Severe haemorrhage and shock

Blood loss from a pelvic fracture can be severe especially if the bleeding is from a torn pelvic or lumbar vessel rather than from the bone itself. The haemorrhage can spread into the retroperitoneal and extraperitoneal spaces and be hidden from view and cause profound loss of circulating blood and shock.

The diagnosis should be suspected in all cases of fractures of the pelvic ring that show the signs of blood loss namely pallor, sweating, restlessness, rapid pulse, hypotension and diminished urinary output. BEWARE OF OVERLOOKING OTHER SITES OF BLOOD LOSS SUCH AS A RUPTURED SPLEEN. Double fractures of the pelvic ring commonly require transfusion. The extent of the haematoma can be gauged by CT scans. Plain radiographs are needed to show if there is any free air in the abdomen but with a haematoma a radiologist may report loss of clarity of the psoas shadow.

TREATMENT

Retro and extraperitoneal haemorrhage by itself is not an indication for operation and may even be a contraindication. Laparotomy is required if:

i. Intraperitoneal damage is obvi-

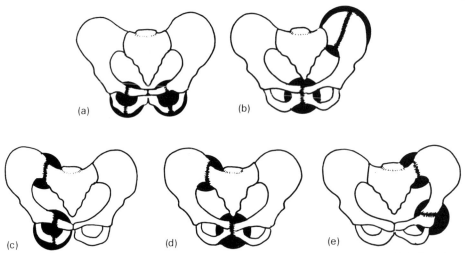

Fig. 3.34 (a), (b), (c), (d) and (e) Some of the many combinations of fractures and dislocations of the pelvic ring. Note that where the ring is broken and displaced significantly at one point there must be a further fracture or dislocation.

ous or there is a positive peritoneal tap for blood.

ii. There are signs of continuing severe haemorrhage after giving multiple units of blood or if rapid transfusions are not sustaining the patient who has been in a G-suit (low pressure suit).

iii. External skeletal fixation is of great value in stabilizing the pelvis and thus controlling bleeding. When peritoneal lavage reveals gross blood, explore the abdomen. If there is no gross blood apply skeletal fixation.

KEY POINTS

a. If possible directly control the point of bleeding.

b. If direct control is not possible ligate the internal iliac artery on the affected side. Both arteries can be ligated if necessary.

c. In less dramatic but persistent bleeding arteriography can identify bleeding points and even allow embolization with occlusive materials through the catheter.

d. A G-suit should be applied over the legs, pelvis and abdomen at an early stage in severely shocked patients. It tends to control blood loss by diverting blood flow. It does restrict breathing and needs to be depressurized every four to six hours for assesment of the skin, the lower limbs and the bleeding problem.

e. Rarely the external iliac vessels are damaged with danger to the viability of the limb. Direct repair or grafting should be

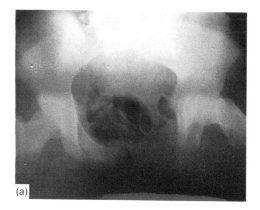

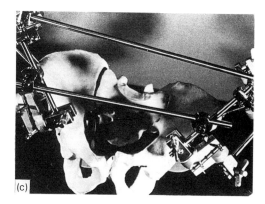

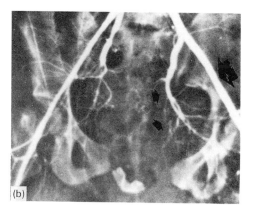

Fig. 3.35 (a) widely displaced disrupted pelvis; (b) there was arterial damage to the external and internal iliac arteries; (c) external fixation as used in this case is shown on a model.

carried out after assessment by angiography.

f.   The pelvic fracture will need reduction and may require immobilization (usually internal or external fixation) where there is vascular injury (Fig. 3.35 (a), (b) and (c)).

TREATMENT

Anti-embolic supporting stockings and early active movements of the lower limbs where possible. Signs of venous thrombosis such as calf pain and swelling call for the use of anti-coagulants but not until 48 hours have elapsed from the time of a major pelvic fracture.

(ii) Thrombosis and thromboembolism

The incidence of deep venous thombosis, thrombophlebitis and pulmonary embolism after pelvic fractures is quite high.

(iii) Damage to pelvic organs and pelvic nerves

Damage to L4, L5, S1, S2 nerve roots and the lumbar plexus occurs occasionally in association with fractures of the pelvis. Where nerve roots are avulsed the outlook is not good.

TREATMENT

Physiotherapy treatment will help muscles recover where the nerves are not permanently damaged.

Up to 40% of displaced fracture of the pelvis are associated with damage to the pelvic or abdominal organs. (The bladder and urethra will be discussed separately.) These injuries are more common in the crushing type of injury seen in industrial accidents. Damage can be to the mesentery or to small or large bowel or the external iliac vessels.

TREATMENT

Recognition and repair.

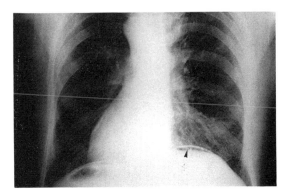

Fig. 3.36 Gas under the diaphragm is a sign of a ruptured viscus.

KEY POINTS

a. **Suspect abdominal and pelvic damage in all displaced pelvic fractures. Be sure to seek expert help.**
b. **All these patients should have a plain radiograph of the abdomen; look for gas under the diaphragm (Fig. 3.36).**
c. **Details of peritoneal taps, exploration and repair of damaged viscera will not be discussed here.**

(iv) Damage to the bladder and urethra

This is the most common serious complication of fractures of the pelvis. Basically any injury that will cause a fracture of the pelvis

can damage the urinary tract. It is therefore wise to assume that all fractures of the pelvis have caused damage to the urinary tract until proven otherwise.

Signs of damage:

1. Haematuria. This is the most common finding. It may simply be due to contusion of the urethral or bladder mucosa. However gross haematuria requires immediate radiological investigation.

   A urethrogram (Fig. 3.37) is indicated where there is frank blood at the urethral meatus and there is bruising in the perineum and scrotum. Wide separation of the symphysis pubis also is an indication for a urethrogram to be carried out prior to any attempt at catheterization.

   A cystogram (Fig. 3.38) will outline the bladder and show if there is any rupture of that organ. It is essential if there is gross haematuria, inability to pass urine, or clear urine is not obtained by a catheter that passes easily.

   An intravenous pyelogram will outline the kidneys and see if they are functioning. It will also outline the bladder and this is important in those cases where it is impossible to pass a catheter and do a retrograde cystogram. Remember that even if a cause is found in the bladder or

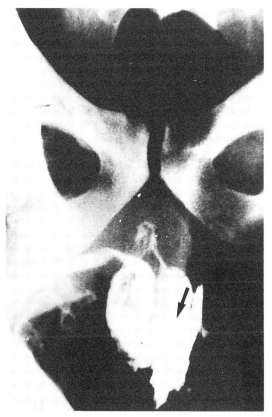

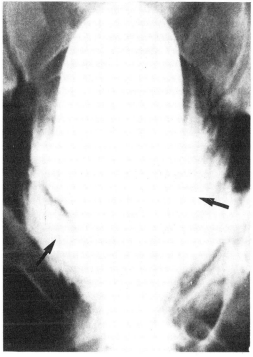

Fig. 3.38 Cystogram showing an extraperitoneal rupture of the bladder.

Fig. 3.37 Urethrogram showing a rupture of the urethra.

urethra for the haematuria, there may also be an injury to the upper genitourinary tract.

2. Inability to pass urine

This may simply be due to the fact that the patient had an empty bladder. However it may also signify a rupture of the urethra or bladder. If urine cannot be passed and there are no external signs of urethral damage (such as blood at the tip of the penis or bruising in the scrotum and perineum), then pass a catheter into the bladder. The presence of clear urine is reassuring but in major pelvic injuries a cystogram should always be done.

3. Pain

In pelvic fractures pain is not a reliable indicator of urinary tract damage.

Types of injury:
These are summarized in Fig 3.37, 3.38 and 3.39.

TREATMENT

Expert help from a urologist is required for all these injuries.

(v) Infection in compound fractures

Compound fractures of the pelvis tend to be very serious injuries and are often combined

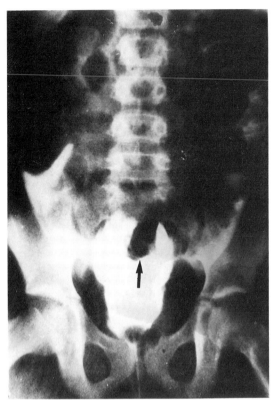

Fig. 3.39 Cystogram showing an intraperitoneal rupture of the bladder.

with vascular damage and damage to the bladder, bowel or rectum. Early mortality is high from uncontrolled haemorrhage, whilst late mortality is often associated with sepsis. Many of these patients will be pedestrians knocked down by a car or industrial accidents. They will often have multiple fractures and head injuries.

TREATMENT

Resuscitation of the patient and restoration of blood volume must be followed by exploration of the wound, repair of the damage if possible, a diverting colostomy if necessary, and drainage of the wounds. If the wounds are contaminated and the fracture unstable then external fixation should be used (Fig. 3.35(c)). Appropriate antibiotics will be necessary.

Retroperitoneal abscess and ischiorectal abscess formation occur at times both in closed and in open fractures of the pelvis when a haematoma in these areas becomes infected. They should be suspected if the patient has high fevers with deterioration of their general condition and a high white cell count. Examination may show an area of localized tenderness. CT scan will define the lesion.

TREATMENT

Ubi pus ubi evacuo – where there is pus let it out. The improvement in the patient's condition will be dramatic. Persistent sinuses will need to be traced to their origin from bowel or bone and the basic problem dealt with. Osteomyelitis of the pelvis is difficult to eradicate, but the same principles of treatment apply as with chronic osteomyelitis elsewhere, the difficulty here being one of access.

KEY POINTS

a. Remove all sequestra and try to leave well vascularized bone.
b. Eliminate any dead space by filling with vascularized tissue such as a muscle graft.
c. Excise any epithelialized sinus.
d. Drain the wound.
e. Give appropriate antibiotics.

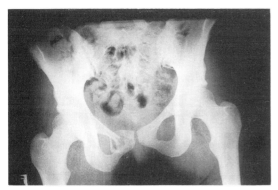

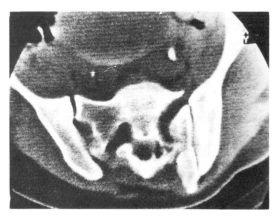

Fig. 3.40 This fracture of the pubic rami will unite with some displacement but this is of no consequence.

Fig. 3.42 Fracture through the sacrum near the sacroiliac joint.

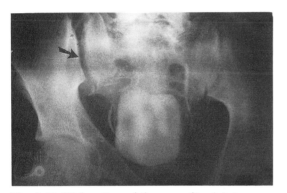

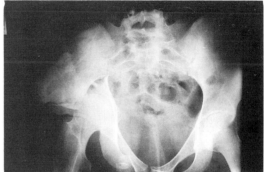

Fig. 3.41 Dislocation of the sacroiliac joint.

Fig. 3.43 Double column fracture of the pelvis with gross distortion and central dislocation of the hip joint.

(vi) Malunion

Some degree of malunion is common in fractures of the pelvis and is of no consequence in many of the isolated fractures (Fig. 3.33 and Fig. 3.40) and in some fractures of the pelvic ring. Persistent dislocation of the sacroiliac joint does cause pain and shortening on the affected side and may also cause malalignment of the hip joint (Figs 3.41 and 3.42).

In female patients the size and shape of the pelvic ring is important if pregnancy occurs. Changes in the size of the pelvic outlet may be an indication for caesarian section (Figs 3.43 and 3.44).

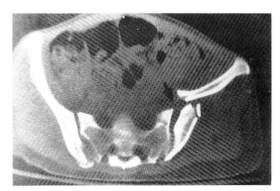

Fig. 3.44 CT scan of a fracture of the ilium and a disrupted sacroiliac joint.

TREATMENT

Reconstructive surgery has become more popular in recent times and many reports of massive reconstructive procedures have been published. The reader is referred to the texts nominated at the end of the chapter.

It must be realized that this type of surgery is difficult and dangerous for the inexperienced. It can involve multiple osteotomies and internal fixation in a crowded and vascular area.

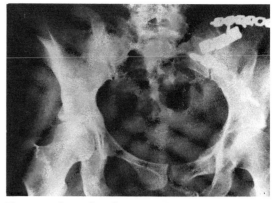

Fig. 3.45 Sacroiliac fusion and pelvic fixation.

(vii) Delayed union and non union

Isolated fractures, avulsion fractures and more rarely some of the pelvic ring fractures can be slow to unite or even not unite. Generally fractures of the pelvis unite readily as the bone is largely cancellous but widely displaced fractures with sacroiliac dislocation sometimes do not unite.

TREATMENT

Displaced fractures of the pelvic ring with sacroiliac dislocation that fail to unite will require reduction (if possible) and fusion using a bone graft and internal fixation of the sacroiliac joint and possibly fixation of the symphysis (Fig. 3.45).

Avulsion fractures with displacement (Fig. 3.46) of the anterior superior spine or the ischial tuberosity can cause pain and loss of power in the thigh muscles. They will require replacement and fixation with limited activity until union occurs.

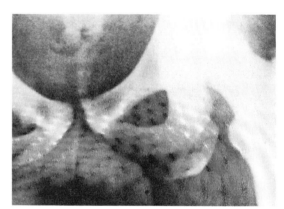

Fig. 3.46 Avulsion fracture of the ischium.

(viii) Damage to the hip joint

Fractures of the pelvis often involve the hip joint directly with resultant damage to the articular surface. There is always corresponding damage to the head of the femur as these fractures occur due to a force transmitted though the femur. This can lead to a traumatic arthritis with disabling pain and stiffness, which can at a later stage require a total hip replacement. It is difficult to prognosticate in individual cases as to the onset of severe traumatic arthritis, but obviously a crack fracture of the ischium that extends into the hip and is undisplaced (Fig. 3.47) is less likely to cause problems than a comminuted fracture that involves the floor and roof of the acetabulum.

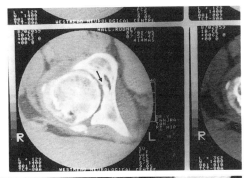

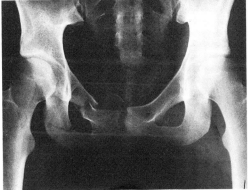

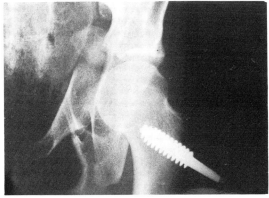

Fig. 3.48 Two fractures of the acetabular floor in lateral traction. Note the gap and the missing piece which are indications for open reduction.

Fig. 3.47 This fracture looks innocent but it does go into the hip joint as shown on the CT scan.

TREATMENT

Since the prognosis is related to the congruity of the acetabulum you should strive to reduce and maintain the normal acetabular shape. For undisplaced fractures simple traction for three weeks and then exercises and graduated activity is advised. For displaced fractures of the medial wall and superior aspect of the acetabulum lateral traction using a Green screw is advised for six weeks (Fig. 3.48) provided reduction is good. If reduction is not good then open reduction should be carried out and the acetabulum reconstructed.

FURTHER READING

Spinal injuries

Anderson, L. D. and D'Alonzo, R. T. (1974) Fractures of the Odontoid Process of the Axis. *J. Bone Joint Surg.*, **56A**, 1663–74.

Bailey, R. W. and Badgley, C. E. (1960) Stabilisation of the Cervical Spine by Anterior Fusion. *J. Bone Joint Surg.*, **42A**, 565–94.

Bohlman, H. H. (1979) Acute Fractures and Dislocations of the Cervical Spine. *J. Bone Joint Surg.*, **61A**, 1119–42.

Holdsworth, F. (1970) Fractures, Dislocations and Fracture Dislocations of the Spine. *J. Bone Joint Surg.*, **52A**, 1534–51.

Kaufer, H. and Hayes, J. T. (1966) Lumbar Fracture–Dislocation. A Study of 21 Cases. *J. Bone Joint Surg.*, **48A**, 712–30.

Pitts, F. W. and Stauffer, E. S. (1970) Spinal Injuries in the Multiple Injury Patient. *Orthop. Clin. North Am.*, **1**, 137–49.

Rennie, W. and Mitchell, N. (1973) Flexion Distraction Fractures of the Thoracolumbar Spine. *J. Bone Joint Surg.*, **55A**, 386–90.

Pelvic fractures

Shatzker, J. and Tile, M. (1987) *The Rationale of Operative Fracture Care*, Springer-Verlag, Berlin.

Tile, M. (1984) *Fractures of the Pelvis and Acetabulum*, Williams and Wilkins, Baltimore.

Letournel, E. and Judet, R. (1981) *Fractures of the Acetabulum*, Springer-Verlag, Berlin.

CHAPTER FOUR

Fractures of the lower limb

4.1 FEMUR

4.1.1 NECK OF THE FEMUR

This is a very common fracture in the over sixty age group and is rare in younger patients. There are some specific differences in management of the complications in the adolescent group and these will be discussed separately.

In the older patient the complications include:

1. Medical and surgical complications of the older patient.
2. Non union and infected non union.
3. Avascular necrosis of the head of the femur.
4. Malunion.
5. Complications after hemiarthroplasty:
   (i) Damage to the sciatic nerve
   (ii) Dislocation of the prosthesis
   (iii) Fracture of the shaft of the femur
   (iv) Infection
   (v) Painful hip joint

In the younger patient the complications include:

1. Non union.
2. Avascular necrosis of the head or neck of the femur.

3. Malunion , Coxa vara.
4. Premature fusion of the femoral capital epiphysis.

Complications

(i) Medical and surgical problems in the older patient

In the older age group (many of these patients are in their seventies and eighties) there can be many medical problems some of which are severe enough to preclude general anaesthesia. Spinal anaesthesia or even regional anaesthesia may be indicated.

In some units fractures of the neck of the femur are treated as surgical emergencies to be operated on at any hour of the day or night. This is not our policy as we believe that a full medical work up will improve the condition of some patients, and show the unlikely survival of others if operative treatment is pursued.

Amongst the common medical problems seen are:

1. Cardiac failure
2. Hypertension and coronary artery disease
3. Respiratory disease
4. Renal failure
5. Anaemia.

Postoperatively there are a number of problems that are common:

1. Chest infections
2. Urinary incontinence and bedsores
3. Wound infection
4. Disorientation
5. Thromboembolic problems
6. Loss of will to get up, walk or even live.

Some of these patients will not survive the first three postoperative weeks in spite of a technically successful operation. It is difficult to always predict those who will survive, but some notice should be taken of the level of activity prior to the fall or injury causing the fracture of the neck of the femur. If a patient has been living at home and has been independent and going out of the house then the chances are good for recovery. Conversely if the patient was bedridden in a nursing home then the outlook is poor.

In some patients the incident that causes the fall may be a minor cerebral vascular incident and this may account for the remarkable deterioration in memory and alertness seen after their admission to hospital.

Thromboembolic phenomena are common after all hip procedures. Many prophylactic treatments have been tried, but all have their problems. Probably the best at this stage is aspirin 600 mg twice daily for three weeks. In patients who have had previous thromboembolic episodes and those that develop them in spite of the aspirin, full anticoagulation therapy with heparin and later Warfarin are necessary.

(ii) Non union and infected non union

Non union of femoral neck fractures is not uncommon. If femoral neck fractures are left untreated almost all complete and displaced fractures will go on to non union (Fig. 4.1). In fractures that have been treated by operation and fixation of various types the incidence is about 10–15%.

Biomechanical factors

The most important factor working against you is the angle of the fracture. Any fracture with an angle of less than 30 degrees to the horizontal axis is basically stable due to the compressive force being greater than the shearing force at the fracture site (Fig. 4.2). This fracture can be fixed and will unite

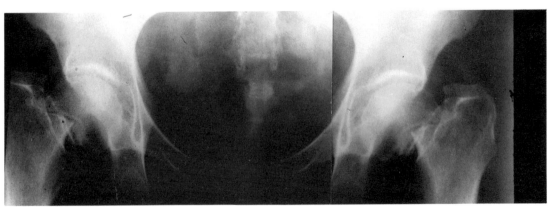

Fig. 4.1 Bilateral untreated fractures of the femoral neck. They will never unite without treatment.

(Pauwels Type 1). If a fractured neck of femur is impacted and in valgus it will unite and does not need fixation.

Non union will not occur.

Compare the situation above to the fracture with an angle of 50° where there is little compressive force and much shearing force. (Pauwels Type 2) (Fig. 4.3). Reduction of the fracture into valgus and internal fixation is indicated. This is much more easily done by open reduction and nailing with compression rather than by blind nailing.

In those cases of fractures of the neck of the femur where the angle subtended by the fracture line to the line of the neck of the femur is 70 degrees or more there is no compressive force only a shearing force at the fracture line (Pauwels Type 3) (Fig. 4.4).

In these cases operative treatment by internal fixation alone will produce a non union as the fixation will either break or cut through the femoral neck (Fig. 4.5).

Operation, if it is to be successful must include a wedge osteotomy in the intertrochanteric region to change the angle of the fracture line and to convert the shearing force into a compressive force (Fig. 4.6)

Non union occurs with:

1. Neglected or unrecognized fractures of the neck of the femur (Fig. 4.7).
2. Poor fixation of the fracture, due mainly to failure to correct the shearing force across the neck of the femur (see above) (Fig. 4.8).

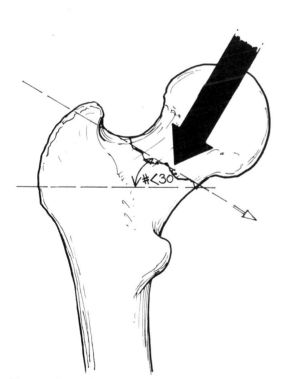
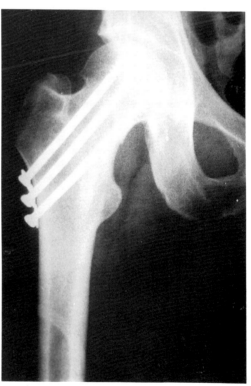

Fig. 4.2 Pauwel's Type 1 fracture. Note the large compressive force with weight bearing and the low shearing force. The fracture does well with pinning in situ.

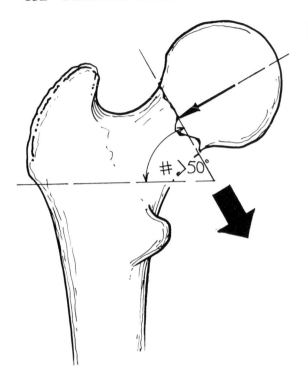

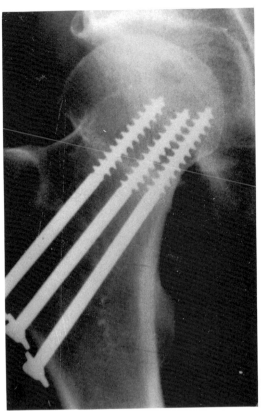

Fig. 4.3 Pauwel's Type 2 fracture. Note the smaller compressive force and the larger shearing force. This fracture needs compression fixation.

3. Avascular necrosis of the head of the femur with absorption of the neck of the femur (Fig. 4.9).
4. Occasionally the bone is so osteoporotic that the fixation whilst initially sound, fails to hold. In some cases the neck of the femur can be paper thin and comminuted (Fig. 4.10).

TREATMENT

The key to successful treatment of these fractures is to carry out the bio- mechanically correct operation. Then the incidence of non union is low. If non union has occurred biomechanical correction and fixation are still necessary provided the bone scan shows a viable head of the femur. If the head is not viable then either a hemiarthroplasty in the elderly frail patient or a total hip replacement in the younger 'elderly' patient is indicated. In the young to middle aged patient another option is to carry out an arthrodesis of the hip.

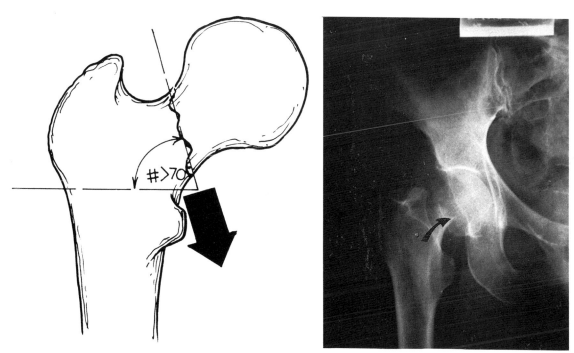

Fig. 4.4 Pauwel's Type 3 fracture. Now there is no compressive force and a large shearing force. This type of fracture does poorly with fixation and requires an osteotomy.

KEY POINTS

a. **Carefully examine the radiographs and decide if the fracture needs simple pinning or if the shearing force needs correction.**

b. **If a corrective osteotomy is needed work out the angle of correction and the size of the wedge to be removed. Draw the radiographs on graph paper to scale and cut out the wedge and check the correction.**

c. **At operation fix the blade of the plate in the neck of the femur before removing the previously marked wedge of bone. The wedge has its base laterally.**

When the femur is brought together after the wedge has been removed the neck and the fracture line have been put into valgus (Fig. 4.6 and Fig. 4.11).

d. **Use a compression jack to bring the osteotomized femur together under compression.**

e. **Bone from the wedge can be used as a bone graft.**

f. **Where avascular necrosis occurs replacement of the femoral head with a prosthesis is indicated in the elderly. In subcapital fractures in frail and elderly patients a hemiarthroplasty is the treatment of choice primarily.**

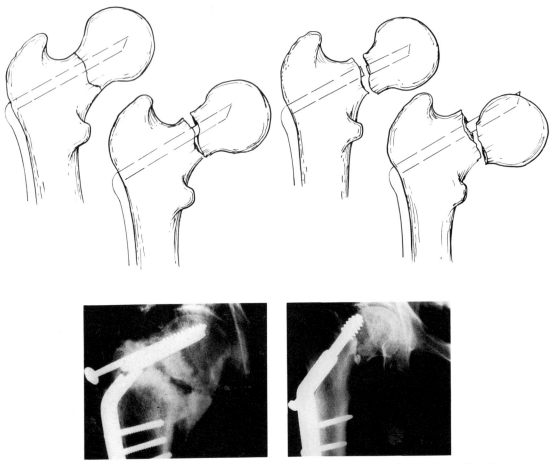

Fig. 4.5 If simple fixation is carried out on a Pauwel's type 3 fracture then the fixation will either break or cut through the bone.

Note:
(i) **A posterior incision (Southern approach) is easier;**
(ii) **Split the gluteus maximus, divide the gemmelli and obturator internus. Identify and protect the sciatic nerve. Open the capsule with a T-shaped incision and remove the head of the femur. Measure the head to help decide the size of prosthesis. Trim the neck of the femur and ream out the medullary cavity with the rasp. Insert the prosthesis and reduce the new head into place. Bone cement can be used to help femoral fixation of the prosthesis (Fig. 4.12(a) and (b)).**

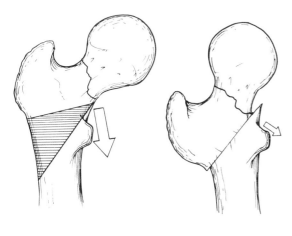

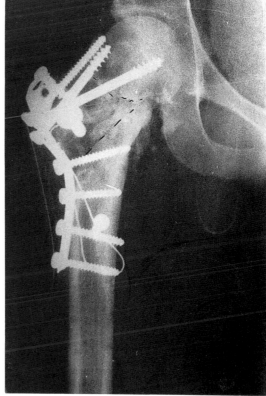

Fig. 4.6 Wedge excision osteotomy converts the shearing force into a compressive force.

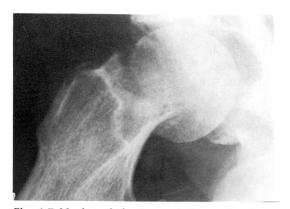

Fig. 4.7 Neglected fracture of the neck of the femur. It will go on to non union.

Infected non union

Occasionally after operation the patient is unlucky enough to develop a wound infection which persists because the neck or head of the femur develops chronic osteomyelitis. Under these circumstances the fracture will not unite, the fixation will become loose (Fig. 4.13) and there will be a chronic discharging sinus.

TREATMENT

In these circumstances the head of the femur becomes a sequestrum. Removal of the internal fixation and excision of the femoral head will be needed to clear up the infection.

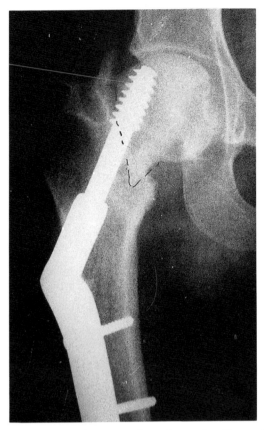

Fig. 4.8 Poor fixation of a Pauwel's Type 3 fracture.

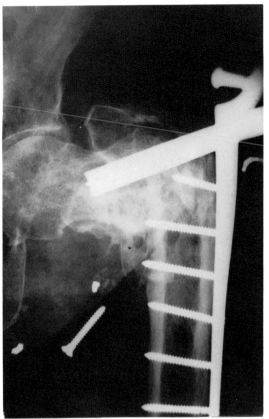

Fig. 4.10 Poor bone strength and bad technique has led to the failure of fixation in this patient.

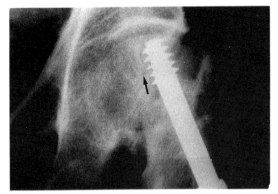

Fig. 4.9 Avascular necrosis of the head of the femur with absorption of the femoral neck.

KEY POINTS

a. **Excision of the femoral head (Girdlestone's operation) (Fig. 4.14(a)) can give a surprisingly good functional result. There is resultant shortening which can be corrected by a built up shoe.**

b. **Because there has been considerable fibrosis associated with the infection, there is not as much shortening as in a non-infected case. After excision of the head of the femur keep the patient in traction for 3–4 weeks.**

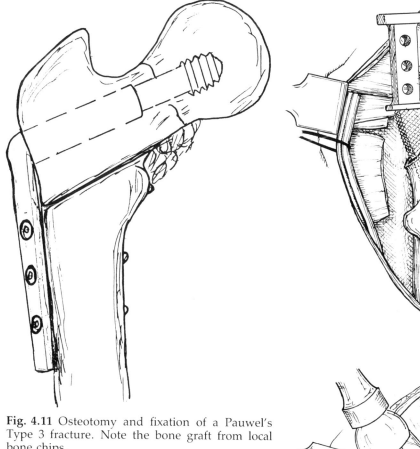

Fig. 4.11 Osteotomy and fixation of a Pauwel's Type 3 fracture. Note the bone graft from local bone chips.

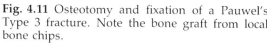

c. If there is too much instability an angulation osteotomy (Milch's operation) improves stability (Fig. 4.14(b)).

Non union in the child or adolescent

Fractures of the neck of the femur have a bad reputation in children and in adolescents. Much of this reputation is associated with the failure to appreciate the difference in bone

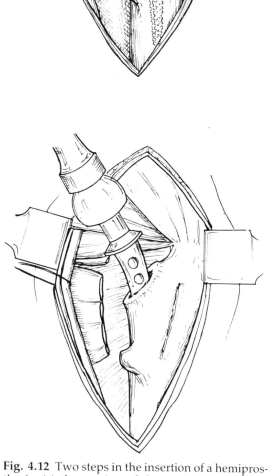

Fig. 4.12 Two steps in the insertion of a hemiprosthesis: (a) the rasping of the medullary cavity to size; (b) the seating of the prosthesis.

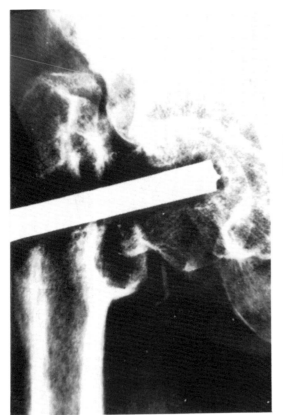

Fig. 4.13 This infected nailing of a fractured neck of femur shows loosening and bone destruction.

TREATMENT

In this age group open reduction and internal fixation using long cancellous lag screws is necessary.

KEY POINTS

a. **This is an urgent operation as the blood supply to the head of the femur can be compromised by the haematoma in the joint.**
b. **Open reduction of the fracture to obtain perfect position is necessary. Closed reduction and pinning will not give a satisfactory result.**
c. **Internal fixation should be with two or three screws which clamp the fracture firmly together and not apart.**
d. **The screws should not go across the epiphyseal plate (Fig. 4.17).**

(iii) Avascular necrosis of the head of the femur

This complication has already been briefly discussed in the adult. It is usually a complication of subcapital fractures and is of course purely a vascular phenomenon. Early signs in adults are increased density of the femoral head due to the loss of blood supply and hence the inability to absorb bone mineral. Later there is loss of sphericity of the head (Fig. 4.18 (a) and (b)) and of course the nuclear scan shows loss of uptake of the radioactive isotope (Fig. 4.19).

In children avascular necrosis can occur in all fracture types including undisplaced fractures but is much more common in fractures that have been displaced and is therefore probably due to a vascular insult at this point.

strength and texture in children and young adults.

At this age the neck of the femur is not the soft almost friable bone we see in the elderly, and our reduction and fixation must take account of this. You cannot use a Trifin (Smith-Petersen) nail (Fig. 4.15) as the bone is too dense to allow it to slide into the neck and it will push the fracture apart.

Reduction is difficult by closed means and most problems in this age group with this fracture arise from failure to reduce the fracture leaving a gap and failure to fix the fracture with the ends firmly opposed (Fig. 4.16).

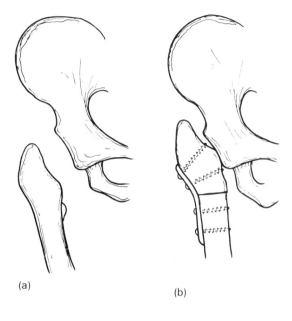

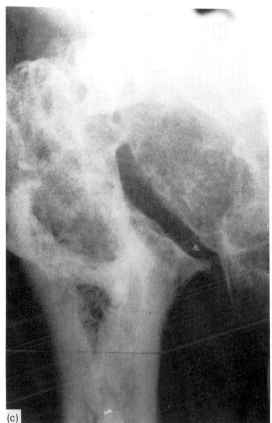

(c)

Fig. 4.14 (a) Girdlestone's operation, excision of the fractured head and neck of the femur; (b) Milch's osteotomy improves stability; (c) Radio-logical view of fixation (Milch's osteotomy).

The incidence in transcervical fractures is probably nearly 50%.

In contrast to adults the onset is slow and it can be twelve to eighteen months before the condition shows. The clinical features are pain and limitation of movement and these may be the earliest features. A nuclear scan will show a decreased uptake as compared to the opposite side. Later a plain radiograph will show increased sclerosis, widening of the joint space, fragmentation and distortion of the femoral head (Fig. 4.20).

This is a disastrous complication in most cases when the whole articular surface is involved. This is unfortunately the most common type of avascular necrosis and the end result is a painful arthritic hip. Much more rarely a small segment of the femoral head or even the neck is involved and the outlook here is good (Fig. 4.21).

TREATMENT

Initially the young patient should be kept non-weight bearing for three to six months to allow for fracture healing and early revascularization. It is believed that the process is prolonged and recently some cases have been treated by the use of an orthosis to contain the head in the acetabulum in rather the same way as in

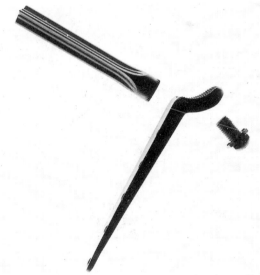

Fig. 4.15 This now superseded nail plate is totally unsuited for children's fractures of the neck of the femur.

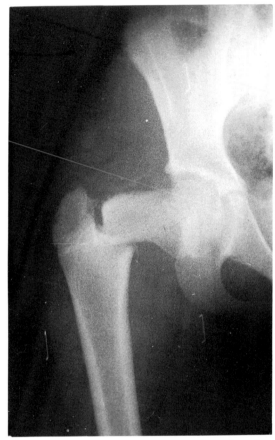

Fig. 4.16 Basal neck fracture in a girl aged twelve. Note the poor position after traction.

the treatment of Perthe's disease (Fig. 4.22). The problem here is that unlike Perthe's, repair is very slow and probably extends over several years.

(iv) Malunion

This is rare in adult fractures of the neck of the femur. If they are not well reduced they do not unite. Either the fixation cuts out or they progress to non union with the fixation holding them apart. Rarely you will see union in marked varus (Fig. 4.23(a)). Some impacted fractures in valgus (Fig. 4.23(b)) will unite in this stable position and give slight leg lengthening, which in itself does not require any treatment.

In children the position is reversed in that malunion is not infrequent, especially if closed reduction is carried out and perfect reduction is not obtained. In addition deformity can occur in varus (Fig. 4.24) or valgus by partial closure of the femoral capital epiphysis.

Total premature closure of the femoral capital epiphysis will give a coxa vara deformity with a small femoral head and a short neck plus overgrowth of the greater trochanter (Fig. 4.25).

At this stage we are uncertain as to why premature epiphyseal closure occurs. Avascular necrosis of the head and neck or pins or screws across the epiphyseal plate may play

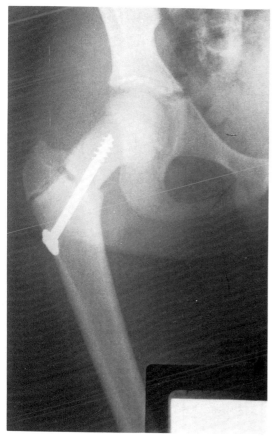

Fig. 4.17 The same fracture as in Fig. 4.16 after open reduction and fixation. Note the failure to correct the varus completely and the use of one screw only giving poor fixation. Fortunately the end result was satisfactory.

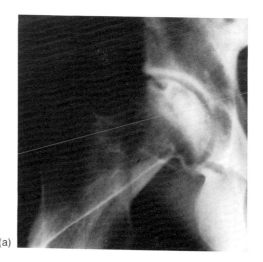
(a)

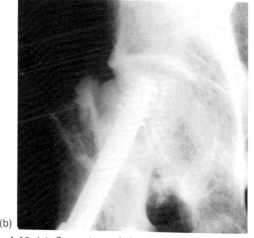
(b)

Fig. 4.18 (a) flattening of the femoral head is an early sign of avascular necrosis; (b) absorption of the neck and distortion of the head of the femur.

their part but in many cases there must be stimulation of the epiphysis by the fracture and repair process.

The effect of the early fusion is to:

1. Cause coxa vara
2. Give a short neck of femur.
3. Cause leg shortening as the femoral capital epiphysis contributes about 15% to leg length. The younger the child the greater the leg length discrepancy.

TREATMENT

Pure coxa vara cries out to be re-aligned by a valgus osteotomy (Fig. 4.26).

In severe cases where there is gross femoral neck shortening and coxa vara a double osteotomy which divides the shaft, neck and

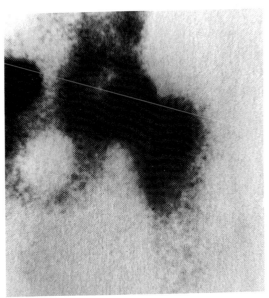

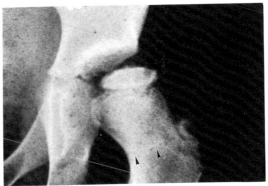

Fig. 4.20 The changes of avascular necrosis, increased sclerosis, widening of the joint space and fragmentation of the head of the femur in a child. Similar changes occur in Perthe's disease.

Fig. 4.19 Nuclear scan showing loss of uptake of radioisotope in the avascular segment.

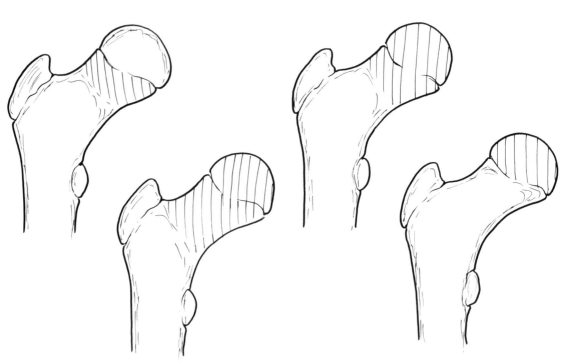

Fig. 4.21 In children avascular changes can occur in different areas of the head and neck of the femur.

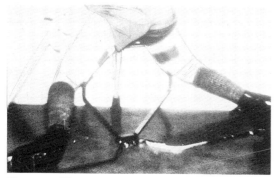

Fig. 4.22 The Toronto splint used for avascular necrosis in children on the same basis as in Perthe's disease.

head into separate components and realigns them is recommended (Fig. 4.27).

> **KEY POINTS**
>
> a. **Insert a Steinman's pin along the axis of the neck of the femur. This will allow you to manipulate the neck into position later.**
> b. **You should carry out two parallel osteotomies, one through the base of the greater**

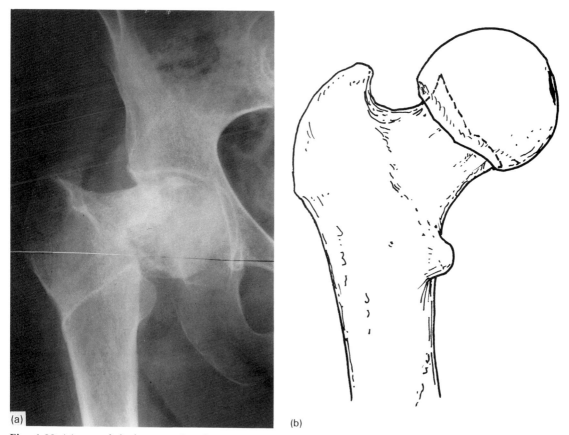

Fig. 4.23 (a) an adult fracture that has united in varus and has avascular changes in the head; (b) fractures that are impacted in valgus are stable if there is a painless range of movement and there will be union without problems.

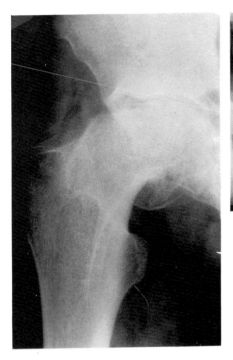
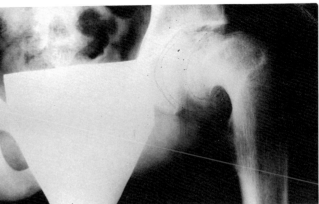

Fig. 4.24 Varus deformity after a fractured neck of the femur in a fourteen year old boy.

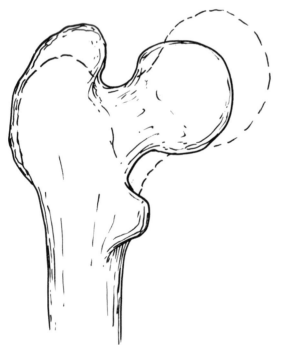

Fig. 4.25 Premature closure of the epiphysis of the femoral neck gives a small head, short neck and an overgrown greater trochanter.

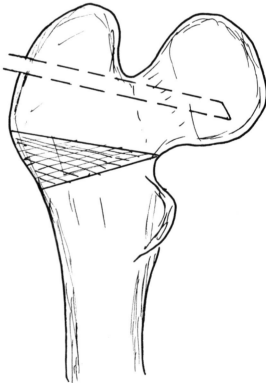

Fig. 4.26 Valgus osteotomy for pure coxa vara.

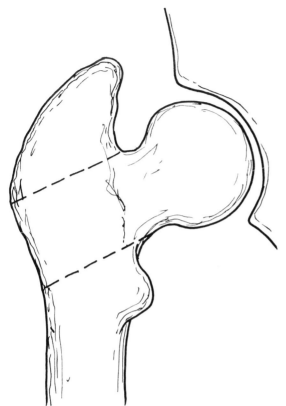

Fig. 4.27 Planning the double osteotomy.

trochanter and the other in the subtrochanteric region.

c. **Redirect the neck of the femur into valgus and move it medially so that the neck becomes longer (Fig. 4.28).**

d. **Mobilize the greater trochanter and bring it down to sit on what was the lateral surface of the femur.**

e. **Fix all the fragments internally with a hook plate, wires and screws (Fig. 4.29).**

(v) Complications after hemiarthroplasty

This excellent operation provides an answer to the problem of the elderly patient with a subcapital fracture of the neck of the femur or an avascular head. It has the virtue of being easy to perform, involves little blood loss and is well tolerated by the old patient. It allows early mobilization (24 h) and immediate weight bearing. There is no danger of avascular necrosis, non union or breakage of the nail or screws. There are some problems:

1. Sciatic nerve damage

The sciatic nerve is a very large and obvious structure that must be identified before the capsule of the hip joint is opened (Fig. 4.30(a) and (b)). Point it out to your assistant and make it the assistant's job to guard the nerve. It is in danger during the opening of the capsule and can also be 'reduced' into the hip joint with the new prosthetic head.

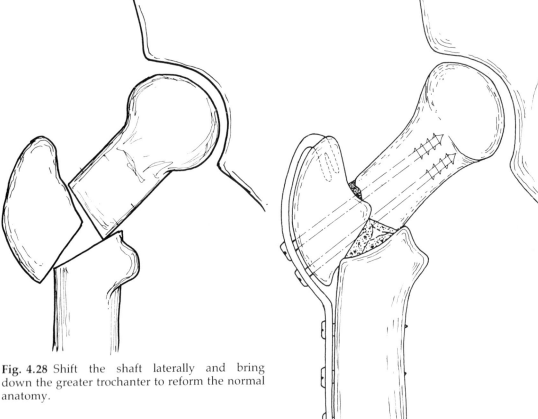

Fig. 4.28 Shift the shaft laterally and bring down the greater trochanter to reform the normal anatomy.

Fig. 4.29 Fixation of the osteotomy may require a hooked plate, wires and screws.

TREATMENT

In most cases the damage is not recognized at the time of injury and the prognosis is poor. Commonly the patient is left with a foot drop and some sensory loss. Further exploration is not warranted in the elderly so that treatment is limited to a toe raising orthosis.

If the damage is recognized at the time operative repair should be undertaken. The results of microsurgical repair are also not good.

2. Dislocation of the prosthesis

Despite capsular repair there is not great stability in the early weeks after a hemiarthroplasty and posterior dislocation of the prosthetic head occurs not infrequently. It occurs when the leg is allowed to internally rotate especially if adducted. This can effectively be prevented by the use of an abduction pillow between the legs for 24–36 hours.

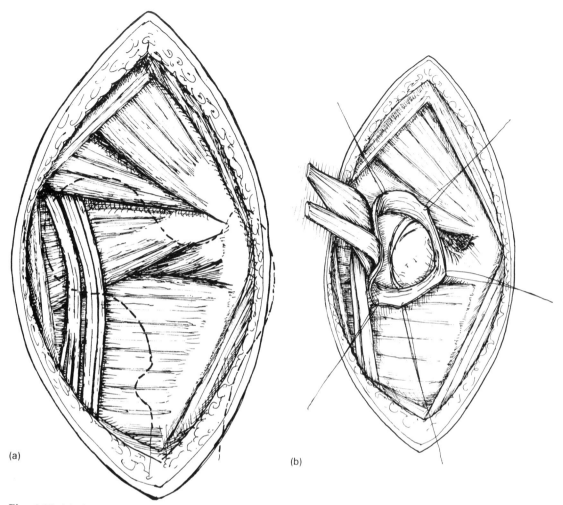

Fig. 4.30 (a) the sciatic nerve should be located after splitting the gluteus maximus as it is in a close posterior relation to the acetabulum; (b) the obturator internus and gemelli should be turned back to protect the nerve.

(a)

(b)

TREATMENT

As soon as the dislocation is diagnosed the prosthesis should be relocated. The diagnosis is obvious clinically as there is shortening and internal rotation of the leg together with pain and limitation of movement. Radiographs will confirm the diagnosis (**Fig. 4.31**).

KEY POINTS

a. Reduction can sometimes be achieved in many cases with intravenous diazepam and pethedine and traction on the leg. If this is unsuccessful then reduction will need to be carried out under a general anaesthetic as follows.

b. Relocation of the head is

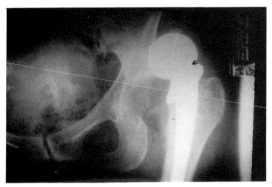

Fig. 4.31 Dislocated Thompson's prosthesis.

achieved by traction on the leg with the knee and hip flexed to ninety degrees. Do not put any rotary stress on the femur or you may end up with a spiral fracture.

c. A second person should apply direct pressure on the prosthetic head, pushing it anteriorly into place.

d. After reduction the patient will need to be kept in traction and external rotation for three weeks to allow the capsule to heal strongly.

e. If the dislocation cannot be reduced by closed means an open reduction will be necessary.

f. If the dislocation recurs then it is probable that the posterior rim of the acetabulum has been crushed and this is the reason for the instability. In these cases there is no alternative to a total hip replacement if the patient is well enough.

3. Fracture of the shaft of the femur

This unfortunate event usually occurs with a sickening crack during attempts to reduce the prosthetic head into the acetabulum. It can also occur during the reaming out of the shaft of the femur. A small number of patients suffer a further injury after they go home and are readmitted with a fracture of the shaft of the femur.

TREATMENT

Crack fractures of the neck or the greater trochanter will require delay in weight bearing. Fractures of the shaft of the femur are best treated by internal fixation at the time of the incident. A long stemmed prosthesis can often be used to provide intra-medullary fixation of a fractured shaft of the femur (Fig. 4.32).

The delayed fracture may be below the level of the prosthesis or involving the prosthesis. The fracture involving the prosthesis may still be adequately splinted by it and may only require bed rest until healing occurs. Those that occur below the fracture site need fixation (Fig. 4.33) if the patient is fit enough or traction if they are not.

4. Infection

As with all operations that involve the use of implants, infection is a major problem when it occurs. Superficial infection is usually not a great problem, and responds to treatment. Deep infection in the elderly may not show the usual toxic response. It should be suspected if there is an increase in pain, nocturnal fever, high sedimentation rate. Aspiration may confirm the diagnosis.

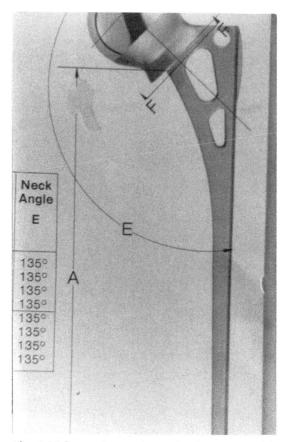

Fig. 4.32 Long stemmed prosthesis may provide medullary fixation of a fracture.

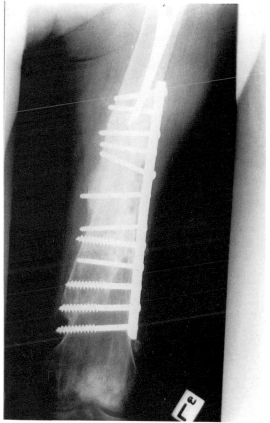

Fig. 4.33 Internal fixation of a fractured femur below the prosthesis.

TREATMENT

Superficial infection will usually respond to drainage and antibiotics.
Deep infections are usually severe and require incision, debridement and drainage under an intravenous antibiotic cover. The mortality rate is high and the chances of retaining the prosthesis are not good.

5. Painful hip joint

There are a number of reasons for this problem:

(a) Basically a metal to bone or a high density polyethylene to bone articulation is not a good one as the coefficient of friction is too high and the bone will wear. Thus if the hemiarthroplasty is carried out in a younger active patient the joint will become painful within three years. On radiograph there is penetration of the head into the acetabular wall (Fig. 4.34).
(b) There can be loosening of the prosthesis in the shaft of the femur. This can be detected by the presence of a rocking track, a zone of translucency rimmed by a sclerotic line (Fig. 4.35).

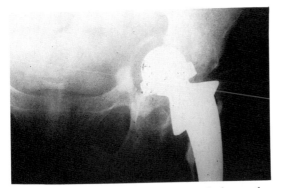

Fig. 4.34 Penetration into the acetabulum of a Monk's prosthesis as usually happens in a metal to bone joint interface with weight bearing.

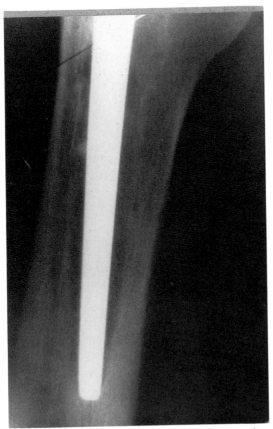

Fig. 4.35 Zone of translucency around a stem is a sign of loosening.

TREATMENT

If the patient is fit enough and the pain is severe enough to warrant further treatment then a total hip replacement is indicated. Hemiarthroplasty is not recommended for young active patients.

4.1.2 SLIPPED UPPER FEMORAL CAPITAL EPIPHYSIS

This condition occurs in young patients, mainly boys between ten and fifteen years old and is characterized by either an acute or a chronic displacement of the femoral capital epiphysis posteriorly and inferiorly (Fig. 4.36). Clinically this causes pain and limping and there is limited internal rotation of the hip and an external rotation deformity of the leg.

There are a number of complications:

1. Failure to recognize the slipping resulting in malunion.
2. Inability to reduce the slip.
3. Failure to fix the epiphysis satisfactorily.
4. Chondrolysis and avascular necrosis.
5. Slipping of the opposite femoral capital epiphysis.

1. Failure to recognize the slipping

Failure to recognize the slipping with subsequent malfusion of the epiphysis can occur if there is a slow slip rather than an acute episode. All children male and female, between the ages of nine to sixteen who have hip or knee pain must be considered to have a slipped upper femoral epiphysis until proven otherwise. The chronic slow slip is usually the one that is missed and often present with medial knee pain and a mild limp.

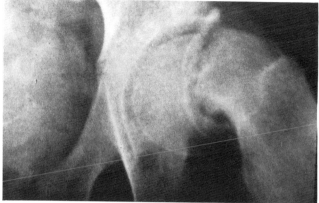
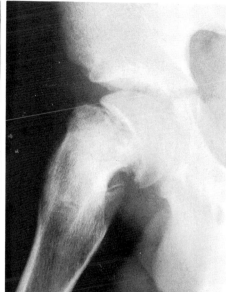

Fig. 4.36 Typical slipped upper femoral epiphysis. Note the posterior and inferior displacement of the epiphysis.

TREATMENT

Recognition of the condition followed by gentle reduction of the slip. If the slip cannot be reduced by gentle reduction then the epiphysis should be pinned in situ.

The femoral capital epiphysis can be likened to the ice cream sitting in a cone (the femoral neck). Turn the radiograph so that the femoral neck is vertical and it becomes obvious if the round ice cream has slipped from the cone (Fig. 4.37).

The various forms of osteotomy will be considered in the next section.

2. Inability to reduce the slipped epiphysis

It is essential to remember that violent or forceful reduction of the displaced epiphysis will lead to vascular damage to the epiphysis. The blood supply to the slipped femoral capital epiphysis is along the posterior border of the neck and this is the tissue that is put under tension during and after reduction.

It is better to accept the slip, especially if it is a long standing one, and plan to do a corrective osteotomy later than to violently get the epiphysis in place only to see it become avascular.

TREATMENT

Gentle manipulation of the hip into internal rotation with the knee and hip flexed should be tried as even in chronic slips the position can occasionally be improved. If it cannot be

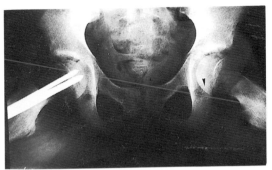

Fig. 4.37 The 'ice cream' is slipping from the cone on the right side. The left side has already been pinned. Slipped epiphyses are often bilateral.

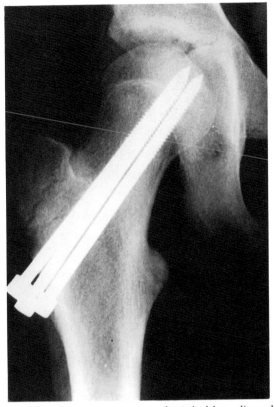

Fig. 4.38 Knowles pins used to hold a slipped epiphysis in situ.

improved the slip should be pinned in situ to prevent any further slip and to obtain fusion of the epiphysis prior to allowing full activities.

Pinning a major slip in situ (Fig. 4.38) will give some shortening and external rotation deformity which can be corrected by transcervical osteotomy or by subtrochanteric osteotomy.

Transcervical osteotomy (Fig 4.39) has a high rate of avascular necrosis even in the best of hands. I favour subtrochanteric osteotomy which should be used to correct gross varus and external rotation. Plan to do the osteotomy two years after the pinning of the epiphysis as you will be amazed at how many cases have spontaneously corrected in this time.

KEY POINTS

a. **Plan the osteotomy to correct the varus and the rotation, draw the details on graph paper (Fig. 4.40).**

b. **Detatch the greater trochanter using a vertical cut.**

c. **Insert the blade of the plate into the neck of the femur before carrying out the osteotomy to correct varus and rotatory deformity.**

d. **Compress the fragments together using the compression jack. Note the greater trochanter has been included in the fixation (Fig. 4.41).**

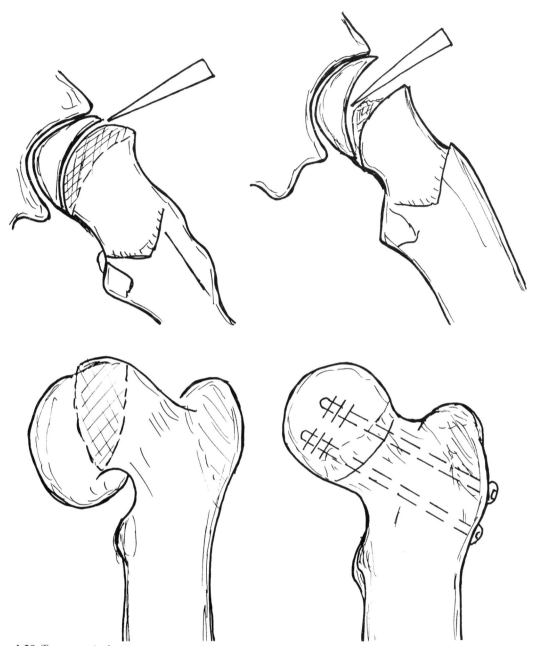

Fig. 4.39 Transcervical osteotomy steps showing excision of the hump and then pinning the epiphysis. There is a high incidence of vascular damage to the epiphysis leading to chondrolysis and arthritis of the hip joint following this operation.

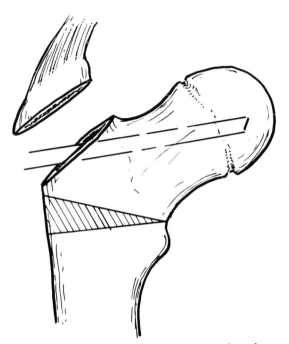

Fig. 4.40 Planning and drawing the subtrochanteric osteotomy. Note the correction can be in three planes.

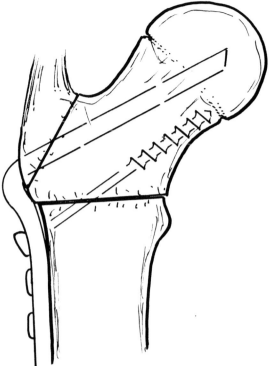

Fig. 4.41 Internal fixation under compression is essential after corrective osteotomy.

4.1.3 PERTROCHANTERIC FRACTURES

These fractures are common in elderly patients and therefore have the same general medical and surgical problems already discussed in fractures of the neck of the femur. They occur more commonly than femoral neck fractures and tend to be in older patients with more osteoporotic bone. In contrast to fractures of the neck of the femur this fracture is through cancellous bone and will unite in about ten to twelve weeks in traction (Fig. 4.42).

Problems associated with keeping the very old patient in traction for this period of time are great and the mortality and morbidity are high so that where the patient is well enough

to take the anaesthetic and operation internal fixation is advised. Most complications with this fracture revolve around the medical condition of the patient or the fixation of the fracture.

They include:

1. Medical problems

(a) Cardiac failure
(b) Hypertension and coronary artery disease
(c) Respiratory problems, chest infections
(d) Anaemia
(e) Renal failure, urinary infection
(f) Disorientation
(g) Bed sores

The patient is of course fully assessed clinically and has appropriate tests carried

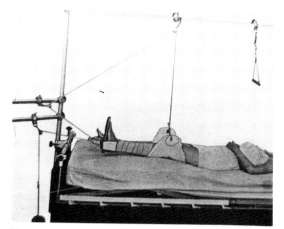

Fig. 4.42 Hamilton Russell traction for a petro-chanteric fracture of the femur.

out. Treatment in hospital prior to operation (such as blood transfusion or digitalization) may improve the patient's condition and allow operation, however the mortality increases with delays over forty eight hours.

2. Fixation problems

(a) Poor bone quality.
(b) Comminution of the fracture.
(c) Failure to appreciate the 'weak point'.
(d) Poor fixation methods.

3. Poor bone quality

Many of these patients have gross osteoporosis and in such patients it is difficult to obtain firm fixation of the implants

TREATMENT

At operation do not tap the screw holes, use cancellous instead of cortical screws and use methyl methacrylate cement to reinforce the bone if necessary.

Comminution of the fracture

The key to stability in this fracture is the medial border. Fig. 4.43 shows the stable type of fracture without comminution of the medial border.

Figure 4.44 shows various types of unstable fractures with comminution of the medial border.

Fractures with posterior and medial comminution are also relatively unstable (Fig. 4.45). They are sometimes known as the 'four part fractures' but may contain three major elements only.

TREATMENT

Stable intertrochanteric fractures represent no problem in fixation with either a sliding screw and plate device, a condylar blade plate and screw, or a 130° plate and screw (Fig. 4.46). The blade of the blade plate should rest on the calcar.

Unstable fractures require careful reduction and fixation of the fracture with reconstitution of the medial border of the femur (Fig. 4.47).

If the medial border cannot be reconstructed then excision of a wedge (removing the comminution) and fixing the head in valgus is recommended (Fig. 4.48 (a) and (b)).

KEY POINTS

a. **The lower osteotomy site is at 45° to the femoral shaft removing 1 cm of the medial border.**
b. **This leaves the proximal fragment with an overhang laterally, but the medial border is now intact and the fracture stable.**

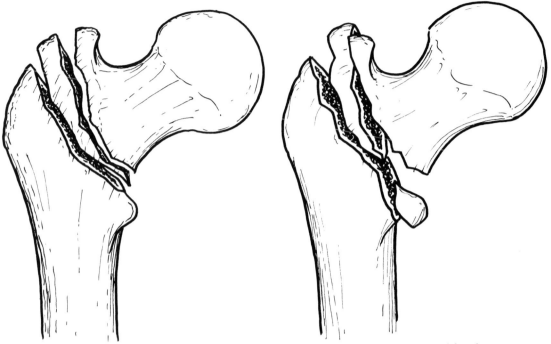

Fig. 4.43 Comminuted pertrochanteric fractures of the femur with a stable medial border.

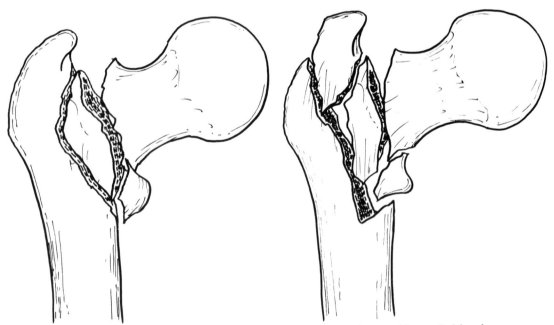

Fig. 4.44 Comminuted pertrochanteric fractures of the femur with unstable medial border.

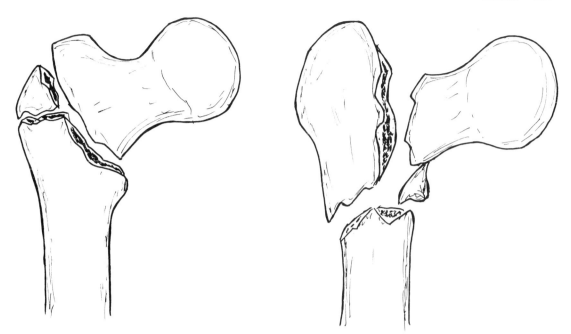

Fig. 4.45 Medial and posterior instability in a pertrochanteric fracture. There is often a vertical split in the piece containing the greater trochanter.

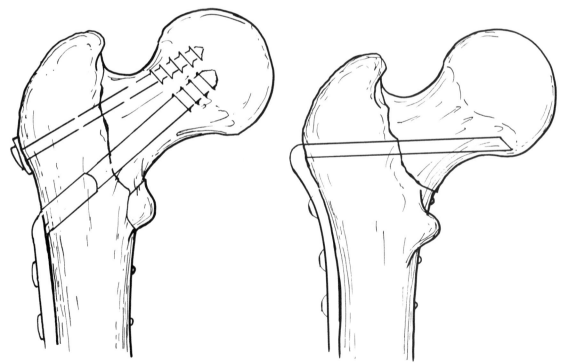

Fig. 4.46 Internal fixation of a stable intertrochanteric fracture.

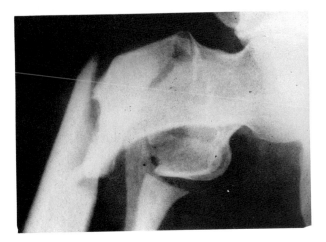

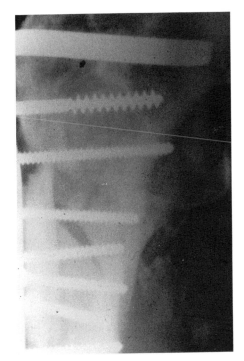

Fig. 4.47 Reconstitution of the medial border and support with a bone graft is essential in fractures with an unstable medial border.

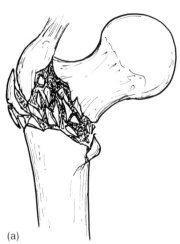

(a)

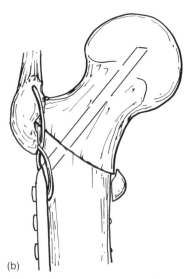

(b)

Fig. 4.48 (a) this type of fracture cannot be reconstructed and needs excision of the fragments; (b) reattachment of the head and neck in valgus to overcome the shortening.

c. **The neck of the femur is in valgus lengthening the leg and compensating for the bone removed.**

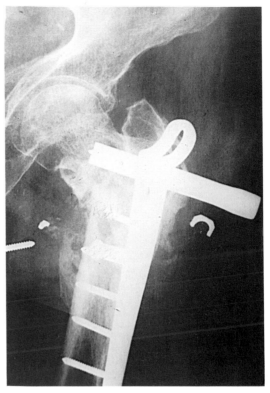

Fig. 4.49 Failure of this system was inevitable.

Failure to appreciate the weak point

As we have already seen the weak point in our fixation is the medial cortex. Frequently we see plates that have broken just below the blade, or bolts that have come undone at the junction of the nail and the plate in a two piece system (Fig. 4.49).

You must appreciate that the medial column must be made intact and protected until it is strong enough to prevent breakage of the fixation. A nail plate system will always break opposite a defect in the medial cortex.

TREATMENT

If a nail plate system has broken then the fracture will go into varus deformity giving shortening and external rotation. The fixation should be replaced and the medial cortical defect repaired and bone grafted (Fig. 4.50) provided the patient is well enough.

Poor choice of fixation

I have already discussed the weak point in the fixed fracture and pointed out the problem at the blade plate junction. Even in relatively stable fractures the blade plate junction is a point of great stress.

It is important then to use fixation implants that will cope with the problem (no implant will cope with a medial cortical defect). Two piece nail and plate systems have a higher failure rate and are not recommended.

The exception to this rule is the Dynamic Hip Screw which when locked in place is certainly as strong as a one piece system and applies some compression at the fracture site.

In recent times Ender's intramedullary flexible nails (Fig. 4.51) have been popular in some centres. These have produced their own set of complications:

1. Failure to obtain fixation.
2. Backing out of the nails from the femur distally and penetration of the femoral head proximally.
3. Supracondylar fracture of the femur.
4. Knee pain
5. Varus deformity and external rotation at the fracture site.

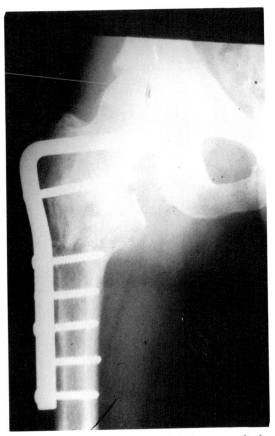

Fig. 4.50 Replating and medial bone graft for previously failed internal fixation.

chanteric fractures. Non union does occur and requires the standard treatment as outlined, namely internal fixation and bone grafting.

It is therefore essential never to leave a defect on the medial cortex opposite the plate. If you do, then the screws will break or pull out, or the plate will break as a result of cyclical loading (Fig. 4.52).

In a fracture in which there is a defect of the medial cortex the cortex should be restored as far as possible and supported by a bone graft. Activity should be limited for six to eight weeks to allow the graft to consolidate before partial weight bearing commences (Fig. 4.53).

TREATMENT

If a plate breaks or screws pull out then reoperation will be necessary using the principles discussed above namely:

1. **Do not leave a defect opposite the plate.**
2. **Buttress the medial cortex with a bone graft.**
3. **Protect the fracture site for six to eight weeks.**

This is a formidable list of complications that has resulted in reoperation in up to 50% of patients treated by this technique. It is not an easy operation to carry out and requires image intensification. Ender's nailing is not recommended.

4.1.4 SUBTROCHANTERIC FRACTURES

These fractures are usually treated by open reduction and internal fixation and have the same problems biomechanically as pertro-

4.1.5 FRACTURES OF THE SHAFT IN CHILDREN

This fracture is one of the more common major fractures. There are many varieties of fracture depending on the level of the lesion, the age of the patient and the amount of comminution present.

In children the complications include:

(i) Complications of Bryant's (Gallows) traction.
(ii) Malunion with shortening.
(iii) Overgrowth of the femur after a fracture.

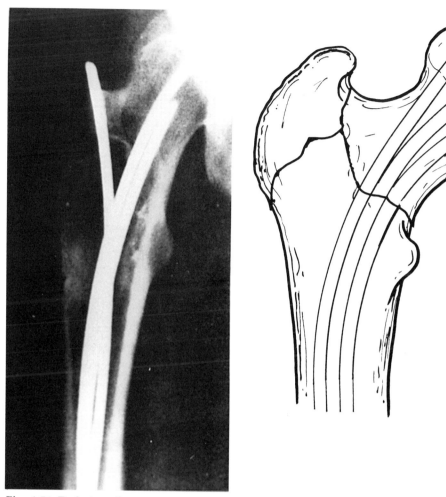

Fig. 4.51 Ender's nails.

(i) Complications of Bryant's (Gallows) traction

Bryant's traction (which was introduced in 1873) is a useful and comfortable way to treat fractures of the shaft of the femur in children of average size below the age of two years (Fig. 4.54).

Problems occur with this type of traction in the older or bigger child as the hip is flexed to 90° and the knee is fully extended, the femoral artery can become stretched and compressed against the inguinal ligament, or the popliteal artery stretched as the child moves and hyperextends the knee. These problems apply to both legs.

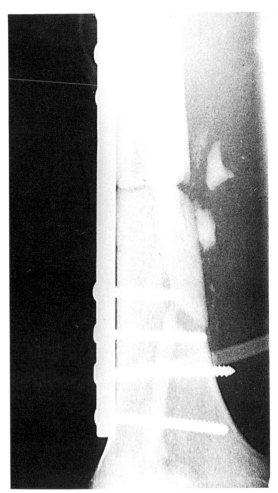

Fig. 4.52 Bony defect opposite the plate will lead to plate breakage.

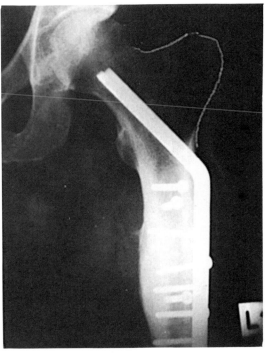

Fig. 4.53 Bone grafting to consolidate the medial cortex.

TREATMENT

This useful and comfortable form of treatment should not be abandoned completely but should be modified by not fully flexing the hips and holding the knees in slight flexion with a padded splint (Fig. 4.55). Bryant's traction should be restricted to children under the age of two who are of not bigger than normal size.

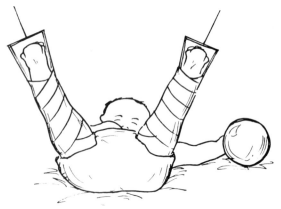

Fig. 4.54 Bryant's traction for fractures of the femur under the age of two.

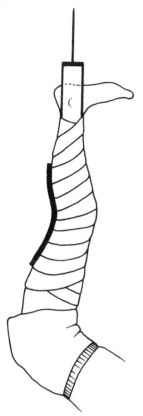

Fig. 4.55 Bryant's traction, a lateral view showing the padded splints to keep the knees slightly flexed.

for 1 cm of shortening and accept 2 cm of shortening if necessary.

3. Where open reduction is carried out overgrowth of 2 cm generally occurs.

Malunion can also occur with angulation and malrotation and this of course is subject to moulding and correction with growth. In the newborn angular deformity of forty five degrees will correct, but this ability to correct depends on the age of the patient and the proximity to the epiphyses at either end of the femur.

The closer the fracture is to the epiphysis, and the younger the child, the quicker and the more complete is the remodelling.

TREATMENT

Persistent deformity can be corrected by osteotomy and fixation but such a procedure should not be carried out for one to two years until the full effects of moulding and growth are known.

(ii) Malunion with shortening

Shortening is a common finding after a fracture of the shaft of the femur in children. Acceptable shortening of 1 cm is unavoidable and in view of the potential for overgrowth discussed below is probably desirable.

A general guide is as follows:

1. Shortening in femoral fractures is permanent over the age of ten years and must be limited to 1 cm.
2. Between the ages of two and ten approximately 1–2 cm of overgrowth occurs in patients treated in traction. You should try

(iii) Overgrowth of the femur after a fracture

Whilst overgrowth is somewhat unpredictable, there is usually some overgrowth in the two to ten year age group. This is usually of the order of 1 cm but can be more, especially if there is initially wide displacement and therefore periosteal stripping.

Open reduction is almost always accompanied by overgrowth of about 2 cm. Intramedullary fixation causes even more overgrowth than plating. The overgrowth appears to occur in the first twelve to eighteen months, and thereafter the growth pattern returns to normal.

TREATMENT

1. **Avoid open operation in diaphyseal fractures in children if possible. Do not use intramedullary fixation.**
2. **Try to leave 1 cm of shortening at the fracture site in most children in the 2–10 age bracket.**
3. **In cases of refracture overgrowth will again be present and rarely may require a leg equalization operation at the end of growth if the discrepancy is greater than 2.5 cm.**

4.1.6 FRACTURES OF THE SHAFT IN ADULTS

This fracture is commonly caused by high energy trauma such as in motor vehicle accidents. There are often a number of soft tissue injuries associated with the fracture requiring specific treatment. The common ones are:

1. Compound wounds in the same leg.
2. Vascular injury in the same leg.
3. Head, abdominal and other injuries and other fractures.

Often the associated injuries dominate the treatment and do not allow the fracture of the femur to be treated ideally.

The common complications of fractures of the femur include:

   (i) Blood loss especially in compound wounds
  (ii) Fat embolism
 (iii) Non union
 (iv) Malunion
       1. Shortening
       2. Angular deformity
       3. Rotary deformity
  (v) Complications related to treatment:
       1. Skin traction
       2. Skeletal traction
       3. Medullary nailing
       4. Plating
       5. Cast bracing
       6. Circlage wiring
       7. External fixation
       8. Infection after internal fixation of the shaft
 (vi) Refracture
(vii) Nerve and vascular injury
(viii) Difficult combined injuries
       1. Fractured shaft and neck of femur
       2. Fractured femur and dislocated hip
       3. Ipsilateral fractured femur and tibia

(i) Blood loss

Fractures of the the femur are deceptive in relation to blood loss. Simple fractures can lose up to three litres of blood into the soft tissues of the thigh and can themselves be responsible for shock and later anaemia.

Blood loss is greater in:
1. Comminuted fractures
2. Compound fractures
3. Combination with other fractures

Beware of attributing the blood loss to the fractured femur without carefully checking to see that there is no other cause, such as a ruptured spleen. Blood loss requires adequate replacement and dealing with the cause of the blood loss.

(ii) Fat embolism

Femoral fractures are the most frequent single fracture associated with fat embolism. Fractures of the tibia and multiple fractures are also associated with this syndrome, which is more common in young adults whose fractures are treated non-operatively.

Fat embolism is a pulmonary complication of injuries to the depots of fat in the long bones by trauma. It is the major cause of respiratory distress syndrome occurring with-

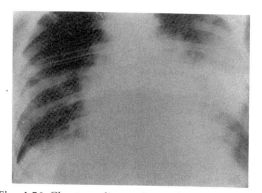

Fig. 4.56 Chest radiograph with cotton wool patches typical of fat embolism.

in the first 72 hours after significant skeletal trauma. Clinical features that dominate are dyspnoea and tachypnoea, profuse bronchial secretions, restlessness and confusion which may rapidly increase and lead to coma, tachycardia, pyrexia and falling arterial blood oxygenation. The chest radiograph has been likened to cotton wool patches or a snow storm (Fig. 4.56). A nuclear scan will differentiate it from pulmonary embolism. Petechial haemorrhages occur in the skin over the anterior chest wall and in the conjunctiva (Fig. 4.57).

The following tests are of value:

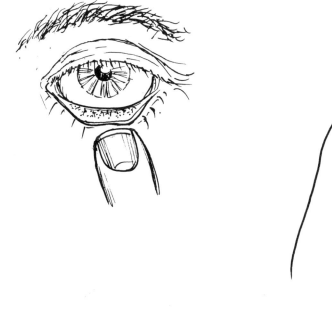

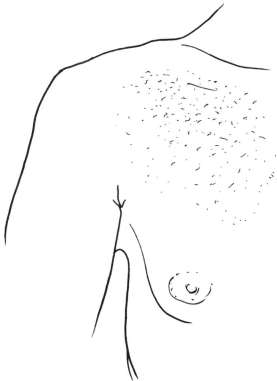

Fig. 4.57 A petechial skin rash over the upper thorax and axilla and in the conjunctiva is seen transiently in fat embolism.

1. Blood gases (PO_2 down)
2. Platelets diminished (less than 150 000/ml is almost diagnostic
3. Fat may be detected in sputum and in the urine

The effect of the fat in the lung is both mechanical and causes a chemical response which results in the destruction of the alveolar architecture and damage to the lung surfactant. This prevents transfer of oxygen to haemoglobin.

TREATMENT

The primary aim of treatment is to reduce the amount of fat embolized from sites of injury and the hypoxaemia associated with the pulmonary deposit of fat.

1. **Gentle handling, proper splinting and careful transporting of all fracture patients.**
2. **Prevention and early treatment of hypovolaemic shock.**
3. **Monitor blood gases early and often.**
4. **Immediate internal fixation of long bone fractures.**
5. **All patients with multiple fractures should have 40% oxygen.**
6. **Assisted respiration with intubation for those patients who cannot maintain reasonable blood oxygen and carbon dioxide levels with oxygen by mask.**
7. **Massive doses of intravenous steroids have been given to help both pulmonary and cerebral problems.**

(iii) Non union

Non union is not rare in fractures of the shaft of the femur and can occur both in cases treated conservatively (Fig. 4.58) or in those managed by operative means.

Conservatively managed fractures go on to non union where the fracture is overdistracted for a long time or where there is muscle interposition or loss of bone (Fig. 4.59).

Operative cases go on to non union when the immobilization is inadequate and holds the fracture apart, or if the leg becomes infected and the fixation fails (Fig. 4.60).

TREATMENT

As with all cases of non union that are not associated with infection the principles are:

1. **Correct any deformity.**
2. **Rigidly fix the fracture.**
3. **Apply a bone graft.**

KEY POINTS

a. **Use a lateral incision.**
b. **Apply a plate under compression (or use an intramedullary nail) after correction of any angulation. The plate should if possible be long enough to allow screws to grip eight cortices each side of the fracture site (i.e. four screws each through two cortices).**
c. **If the fracture is in the subtrochanteric region or near the femoral condyles use a blade plate.**
d. **Use cancellous bone from the iliac crest opposite and around the fracture site and in any defect that comminution may have caused.**

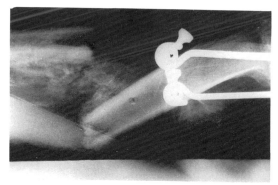

Fig. 4.58 Non union of a fractured femur treated in skeletal traction. Note the posterior displacement and angulation.

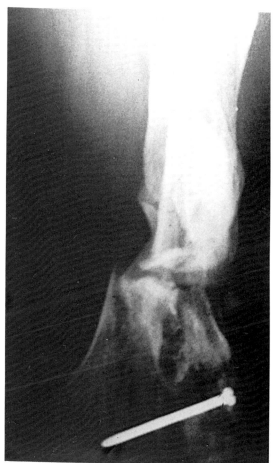

Fig. 4.60 Non union of a compound fracture of the distal end of the femur. Osteomyelitis developed.

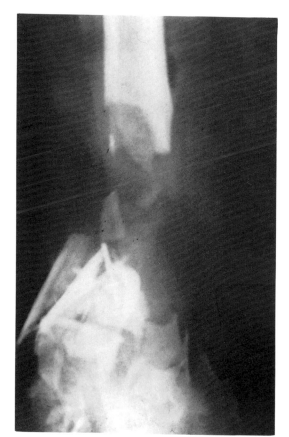

Fig. 4.59 Non union due to missing bone in a grossly comminuted compound fracture of the distal third of the femur.

(iv) Malunion

Malunion in the form of shortening, angular deformity or malrotation (or combinations of these) is common in fractures of the femur particularly in those treated conservatively in traction or in plaster.

1. Shortening

Whilst it is the aim in young children to have 1 cm of shortening at the fracture site, in adults the aim must be to have full length and perfect alignment as adults have virtually no power to remodel or correct any deformity.

TREATMENT

Shortening of greater than 2.5 cm will require a build up of the shoe and usually justifies a leg equalization operation.

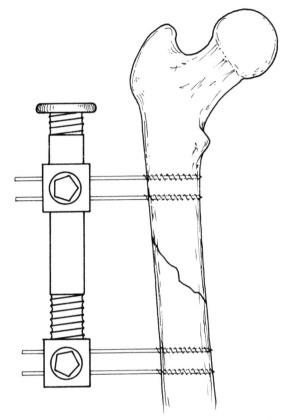

Fig. 4.61 Wagner leg lengthening device can be used to distract and hold a shortened femur.

┌─── **KEY POINTS** ───────────

a. **It is difficult but by no means impossible to regain length in a limb with shortening in a recently fractured femur as the nerves and blood vessels are not stretched by being restored to their normal length.**

b. **It is usually easier to regain the length at the fracture site by undoing the fracture and then stretching the femur to length with the aid of a distractor (Figs 4.61 and 4.62).**

c. **Having obtained full length be sure that the rotation of the fragments is correct and then plate the fracture and fill any defect and the area of the fracture with cancellous bone from the iliac crest.**

d. **Occasionally in a tall person it is better to shorten the opposite leg by removing a length of bone from the subtrochanteric region and applying an angle plate under compression (Fig. 4.63).**

2. Angular deformity

Lateral, posterior and medial bowing produce deformity that is noticeable and causes problems at the knee by altering the weight bearing line. Of all the angular deformities the least noticeable and most benign is a small amount of anterior bowing.

TREATMENT

Angular deformity can be corrected fully by osteotomy and fixation, carefully filling any defect with a bone graft. The fixation can be either by plate and screws under compression or by intramedullary nailing (Fig. 4.64(a) and (b)).

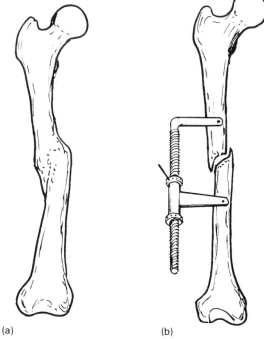

(a)   (b)

Fig. 4.62 (a) and (b) Femoral distractor allows powerful distraction at the time of operation.

3. Rotary deformity

This deformity is quite common and makes the patient very unhappy. Each step they take is a reminder that the foot on the injured side now points in the wrong direction. The deformity can occur both in fractures treated by operation and conservatively. Intramedullary nailing using an 'unlocked' straight nail without reaming does not control rotation.

TREATMENT

A rotation osteotomy with fixation will correct the deformity.

```
┌─ KEY POINTS ─────────────────┐
```

KEY POINTS

a. **It is best to correct the deformity at the fracture site.**
b. **As it is difficult to judge the degree of correction use vertical marks on the shaft of the femur to indicate to you the amount of correction.**
c. **If an intramedullary rod is being used add an anti-rotation plate or screws interlocking into the nail (Fig. 4.65).**

(v) Complications related to treatment

1. Skin traction

Skin traction is an unsatisfactory way of trying to reduce and maintain alignment in a displaced fracture of the femoral shaft in adults.

The problems are:

(a) It is impossible to maintain a pull of more than 3–4 kg for any length of time without the traction slipping or the skin tearing.
(b) It is very uncomfortable for the patient.
(c) If it is applied on the lateral side above the knee then a nerve palsy (which may not recover) involving the lateral popliteal nerve may result from traction on the nerve. The end result may be a foot drop. Skin traction must not go above the head of the fibula laterally.
(d) It is ineffective if there is shortening.

2. Skeletal traction

This can be by a thick threaded pin through the tibia (such as a Denham pin) at the level of the tibial tuberosity or by a thinner pin through the distal end of the femur.

The problems are:

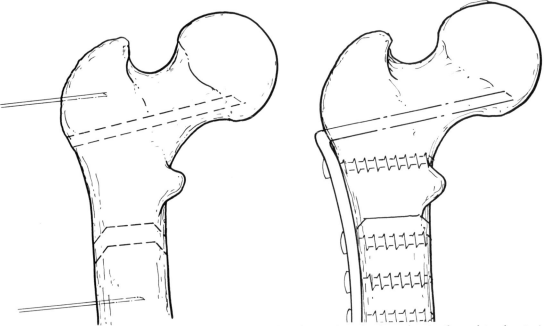

Fig. 4.63 Leg length discrepancy can be overcome by shortening the long leg in the subtrochanteric region. This involves an operation on the 'good' leg.

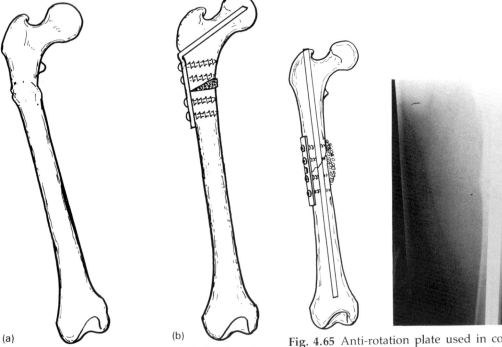

(a)

(b)

Fig. 4.64 (a) and (b) Osteotomy and fixation for angular deformity of the femur.

Fig. 4.65 Anti-rotation plate used in conjunction with an intramedullary nail. Locking the nail with transfixion screws also prevents rotation.

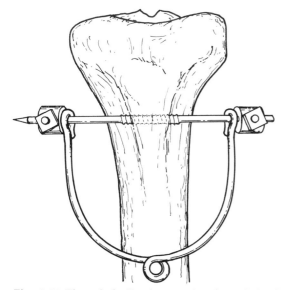

Fig. 4.66 Threaded Denham pin for skeletal traction.

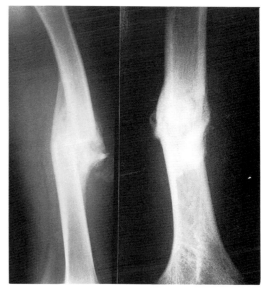

Fig. 4.67 Residual shortening, angulation and rotation after conservative management of a fracture of the shaft of the femur.

(a) Slipping of the pin. A smooth pin without threads will often be loose after a few days especially if the pin has been inserted with a power drill causing excess heat and bone necrosis. Use a threaded pin such as a Denham pin, drill a hole with a drill bit and then insert the pin (Fig. 4.66).

(b) Infection at the pin site. This often occurs if a loose pin is left in situ especially if there has been bone necrosis. Generally the infection is slight and relocation of the pin allows healing. Occasionally a ring sequestrum appears and requires removal.

(c) Malunion to some degree is common in fractures of the femur treated in traction. Shortening and posterior angulation are the common deformities.(Fig. 4.67). In most centres operative treatment has superseded traction as the primary treat-ment of displaced fractures of the femur so as to avoid residual deformity and pro-longed hospitalization (Fig. 4.68).

(d) Traction through the distal end of the femur in the 90/90 position (Fig. 4.69) is less popular but is more direct and more effective and not at all likely to cause knee problems.

(e) All forms of traction run the risk of over distraction in an effort to control align-ment. Persistent over distraction is com-monly associated with non union as discussed previously (Fig. 4.70).

3. Medullary nailing

Fractures of the femur are commonly treated by medullary nailing and while the results are excellent there are many possible prob-lems. They include:

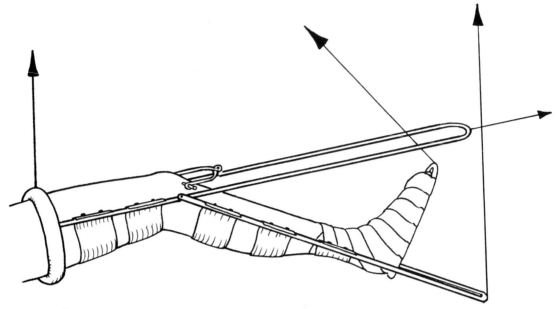

Fig. 4.68 Skeletal traction in a Thomas splint with a Pearson knee flexion piece.

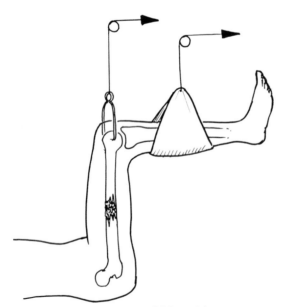

Fig. 4.69 Traction in the 90/90 position.

(a) Fracture unsuitable for nailing
(b) Technical problems
    (i) Burst femur
    (ii) Stuck nail
    (iii) Nail too long, too short, too thin
    (iv) Difficulties with locking the nail
(c) Non union and broken nails
(d) Infection after medullary nailing

(a) Fractures unsuitable for nailing   Wrong selection of patient for nailing: Not all fractures of the femur are suitable for nailing. Essentially the nail needs to splint the femur internally and will not do this at the proximal or distal ends. The ideal fracture for nailing is in the isthmus area in adults. If it does not grip then it must be locked by cross screws and weight bearing delayed. Locking with cross screws prevents rotation.

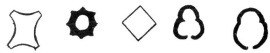

Fig. 4.71 Some medullary nails commonly used.

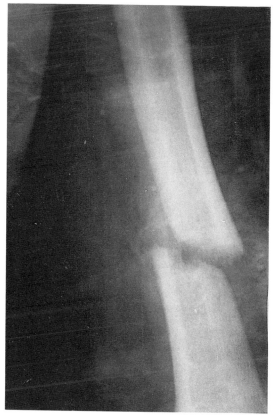

Fig. 4.70 Overdistraction will lead to non union.

Open or closed nailing? Closed nailing requires skill, image intensification, the use of a fracture table and some exposure of the surgeon and patient to radiation. Open reduction with a small incision to guide the rod through the fracture site and hold the reduction is quick, simple and does not require a fracture table or radiation. Having done it both ways I strongly favour the open method.

(b) Technical problems   There are currently many types of medullary nail ranging from the original straight Kuntscher nail to the anteriorly bowed AO nail with its cloverleaf cross section and conical bolt for insertion and removal of the nail (Fig. 4.71).

The Huckstep nail is square and has a compression jig as well as locking screws (Fig. 4.72), while the the Hansen Street nail is like a self broaching I beam. The Schneider nail is diamond shaped and Enders nails are thin flexible rods (Fig. 4.51). There are many others.

Other differences include locking screws at one or both ends to overcome the lack of rotational stability and to maintain length (Fig 4.73).

The isthmus of the shaft of the femur should be reamed to obtain better fixation and improved rotational stability as advocated by Kuntscher and the A O group (Fig. 4.74 (a), (b), (c) and (d)).

(i) Burst femur   This disaster can occur when there is an undetected vertical crack in the femur as well as a horizontal fracture. An intramedullary nail exerts an enormous force on the circumference of the femur. Even half a millimetre increase in size increases the force dramatically and may split the femur. Avoid trouble by accurate reaming and using the nail of the same diameter as reamed.

TREATMENT

The problem will need to be tackled case by case as each fracture will be comminuted by the bursting in a different way. It may be possible to hold the fracture with circlage wires for six weeks or so whilst leaving the nail in situ. Sometimes it is better to abandon the nailing and hold the fractures with a plate and screws and

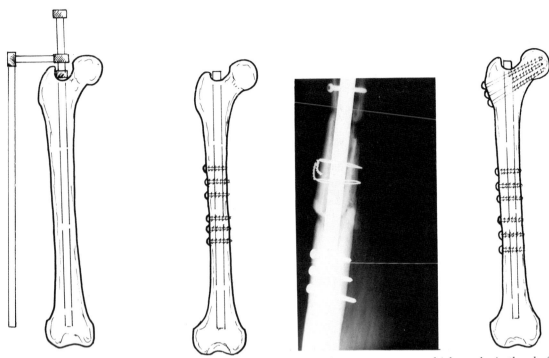

Fig. 4.72 The compression jig and Huckstep nail with the locking cross screws which can be in the shaft and/or the neck of the femur.

a bone graft (Fig. 4.75). One other possibility is to lock the nail with cross screws at both ends.

(ii) Stuck nail   This situation occurs when a nail of too large a diameter is inserted and can neither progress forward nor be removed. It tends to occur when the nail is inserted without reaming and so a nail that seems initially to be fitting well jams at a tight spot.

A similar situation can occur whilst reaming and the reamer gets stuck.

Occasionally a nail that has been in place for a number of years seems to have bone grow all around it and proves difficult to remove.

TREATMENT

Most removing jigs consist of a hook to fit into the eye of the nail (or a conical bolt) and a sliding ram. These are inadequate in this situation.

┌─ **KEY POINTS** ─────────
│
│ **a. Sterilize a pair of vice grip**
│   **pliers and apply this to the nail.**
│   **If there is an eye in the nail**
│   **apply the vice grips below the**
│   **eye and put a dissector through**
│   **the hole.**
│ **b. Use a mallet to hit against the**

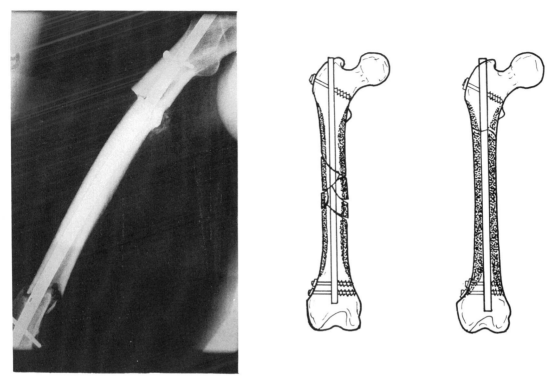

Fig. 4.73 Locking screws in the proximal and distal femur prevent rotation and maintain length.

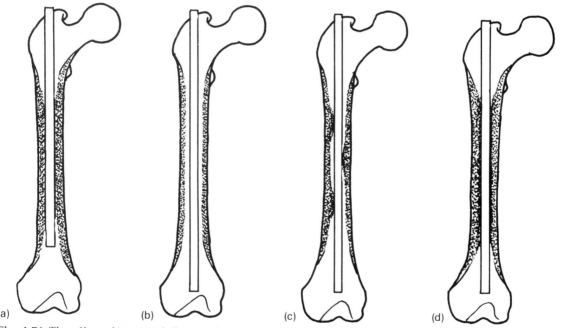

(a)   (b)   (c)   (d)

Fig. 4.74 The effect of intramedullary nails that are (a) too short; (b) too thin; (c) without reaming; (d) as it should be done, reamed to the width of the nail so that there is firm fixation along a wide area.

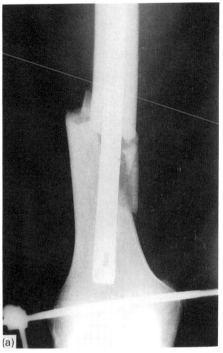
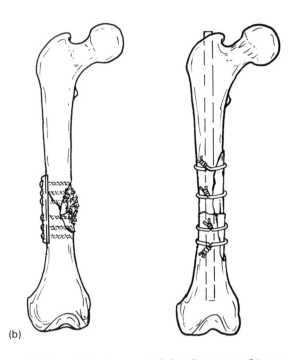

Fig. 4.75 (a) burst femur. Note the skeletal traction applied has still not corrected the alignment. (b) two ways of handling the burst femur, wiring around the nail and reconstruction with a plate, screws and bone grafting.

pliers which are compressing the nail. In between blows try to rotate the nail (Fig. 4.76).

c. A similar arrangement can be made on the nobbed guide rod when a reamer gets stuck (Fig. 4.77).

d. There are times when these manoeuvres will not shift a stuck nail. Then there is no alternative to making a vertical saw cut in the femur to release the nail.

(iii) Nail too short, too thin, too long The ideal intramedullary nail is one that is the correct circumference and grips the femur above and below the fracture site. The straight nail used unreamed depends on three point fixation to hold the fracture, and so the longer the nail goes distally the better. When reaming is used the nail length is not so critical and it does not matter if the nail ends several centimetres above the distal cortex (Figs 4.74).

If a nail is too thin it will not hold the fracture and there is a strong possiblity that the nail will bend or break (Fig. 4.78) and the fracture will go onto malunion or non union.

Obviously you should avoid penetration of the knee joint.

Try to avoid having the nail protruding proximally as this causes pain and discomfort to the patient.

(iv) Difficulties with interlocking nails Interlocking nails have recently become popular and have improved the stability of medul-

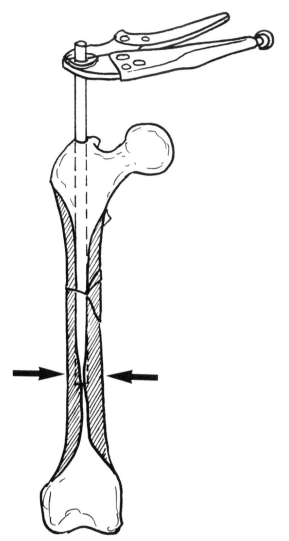

Fig. 4.76 How to remove a stuck nail.

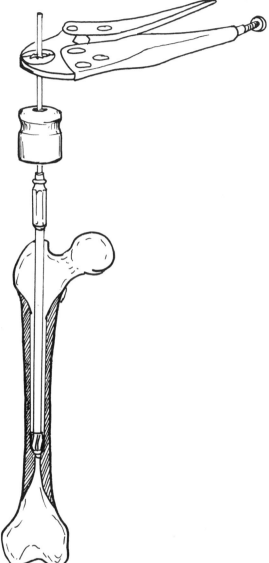

Fig. 4.77 How to remove a stuck guide rod and reamer.

lary nailing where the shaft is not reamed. Their use allows length to be maintained and rotationally unstable fractures to be nailed, with early mobilization. In addition fractures distal to the isthmus can now be held by a combination of the nail and the locking screws. Good results have been reported. It is however technically difficult and in my opinion does not replace the standard intramedullary nail with reaming for the trans-

verse or oblique fracture in the middle third. It is an alternative to plating and a bone graft for the comminuted fracture of the shaft of the femur.

The following are a selection of the complications.

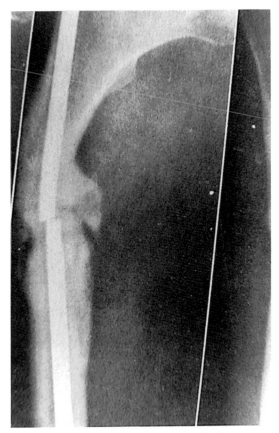

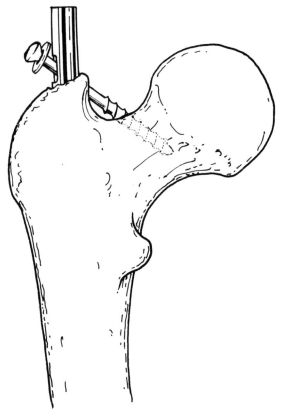

Fig. 4.78 Broken Kuntscher nail which was too small.

Fig. 4.79 Proximal screw cut out associated with a nail that is not inserted fully.

1. The position of the locking screws is dictated by the length of the nail, thus a nail which is too long may have the proximal screw too high (such as in the neck of the femur) and it will cut out (Fig. 4.79). If the distal holes are too far down the locking pins can protrude subcutaneously (Fig. 4.80).

TREATMENT

If the proximal fixation screw cuts out and shortening results then the choice is between renailing with a shorter locked nail or using a plate and a graft. Shortening and malrotation should not be tolerated.

2. It is technically difficult to drill the hole in the distal femur so as to correspond with the hole in the nail. Various jigs tend to be inaccurate distally and image intensification is necessary. One technique is shown in Fig. 4.81. The basis is to align the holes in the nail so that they are symmetrical on the image intensifier. Then place the drill in the hole. All techniques involve some exposure of the surgeon's hands to radiation.

3. It is possible to miss the nail with the

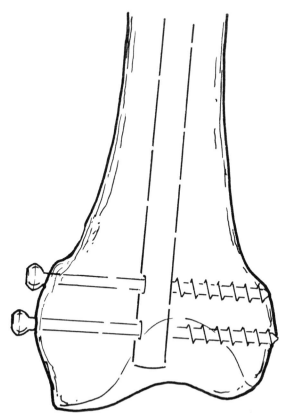

Fig. 4.80 This nail is too long so that the screws will be subcutaneous.

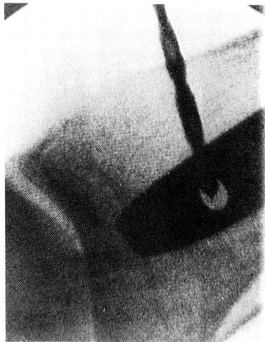

Fig. 4.81 Freehand method of drilling the hole for the cross screw distally. Firstly line up the opposite holes in the radiograph beam and then place the drill in the hole.

screw both proximally and distally (Fig. 4.82).

TREATMENT

If this occurs then resite the screw through the hole in the nail under image intensification or move to an alternate method of fixation.

4. Some femoral fractures have been locked with screws in an angulated and shortened position or in malrotation (Fig. 4.83). At operation on a fracture table it can be difficult to assess leg length.

TREATMENT

It is better to abandon locked nailing if there is significant deformity and do what was probably better in the first place namely, reconstruction of the femur with plating and grafting.

5. While non union is not common, grossly comminuted fractures where there is no bone contact may not go on to bone union and the nail will break (Fig. 4.84).

TREATMENT

This will depend on the type of fracture. It may be suitable for a reamed

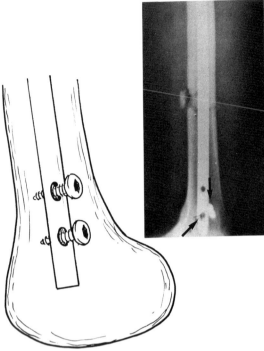

Fig. 4.82 Care needs to be taken to be sure the cross screw goes through the nail.

nail and a bone graft, but it is more likely to be a comminuted fracture that requires reconstruction over a plate and extensive bone grafting.

(c) Non union and broken nails A broken nail is an infrequent but difficult complication. It is usually associated with non union (Fig. 4.85).

TREATMENT

The non union calls for treatment with better fixation and a bone graft after removal of the two pieces of the nail. The proximal piece is easy, the distal half is the problem.

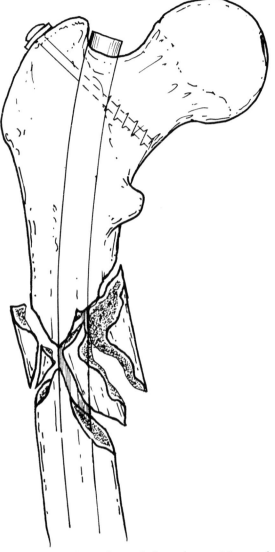

Fig. 4.83 Locking the nail fixes the position and you will need to avoid rotary deformity and shortening in comminuted fractures.

KEY POINTS

a. **A jig is available which can be threaded down the medullary canal and will catch on the distal end of the nail and allow its withdrawal.**

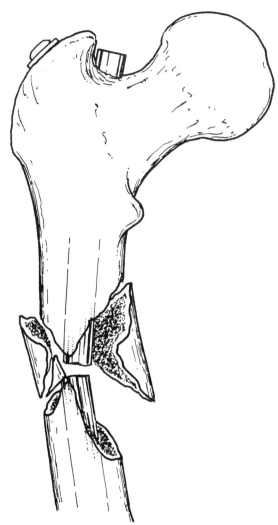

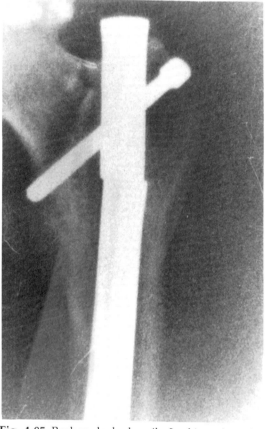

Fig. 4.85 Broken locked nail. Locking does increase the chances of breakage if the nail is loose.

Fig. 4.84 Comminuted fractures may also go on to non union and nail breakage.

b. Alternatively a small window can be made in the femur distally and the nail can be pushed out from below.

(d) Infection after medullary nailing Infection after internal fixation is discussed below and the principles are the same in infected nailing.

1. Leave the nail in situ while it is providing stability.
2. Provide drainage and suitable antibiotics.
3. Persistent drainage in the absence of fulminating infection is not an indication for removal of the nail.
4. If possible leave the nail in place until union occurs and the fracture has consolidated.
5. If the nail is loose remove the nail and stabilize the fracture with external fixation.

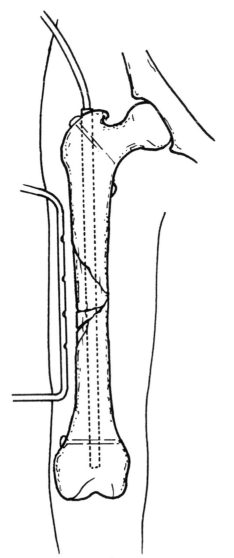

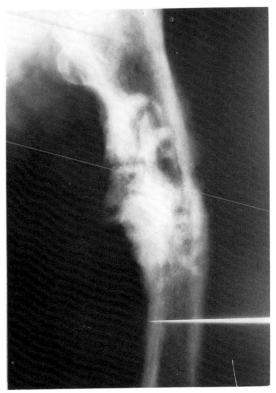

Fig. 4.87 Radiograph showing residual osteomyelitis after medullary nailing.

Fig. 4.86 Suction drainage subperiosteally and in the medullary cavity for a severe infection in a nailed femur.

6. In fulminating infections a suction irrigation system in the medullary canal can be helpful (Fig. 4.86).
7. Residual osteomyelitis is treated by removal of dead bone and drainage until healing occurs (Fig. 4.87).

4. Plating

There is no doubt that biomechanically, plating is inferior as a method of fixation of fractures of the femur when compared to intramedullary nailing. However it does have some advantages and is often my preferred method of treatment.

Advantages

1. Comminuted fractures can be accurately reduced with interfragmentary compression and stability will be restored.
2. Fractures above and below the isthmus can be maintained (Fig. 4.88) and there is full control of rotation.

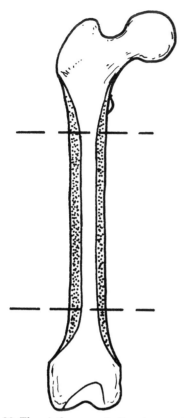

Fig. 4.88 The isthmus of the femur is ideally suited for nailing in non-comminuted fractures. Above and below the isthmus the nail will need to be locked or plating carried out.

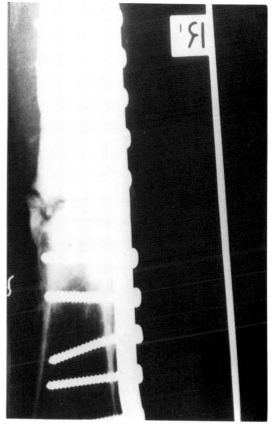

Fig. 4.89 Bone grafting is important where fractures of the femur are plated.

3. The fracture can be easily supported by a bone graft (Fig. 4.89).

Complications of plating   Plate breakage is almost invariably due to poor technique, the most common failing being due to a defect being left in the cortex opposite the plate (Fig. 4.90), instead of being filled in with bone graft.

Another common technical fault leading to plate breakage is to plate the fracture apart instead of compressing it together (Fig. 4.91). Unrestricted activity and early weight bearing may cause the fixation system to fail.

TREATMENT

Treatment of plate breakage
   Reoperation and replating will be necessary with a bone graft added to the fracture site (especially opposite the site of plate breakage). Protect the leg from the stress of weight bearing until the bone graft starts to consolidate in about six weeks (Fig. 4.92).

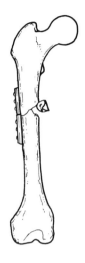

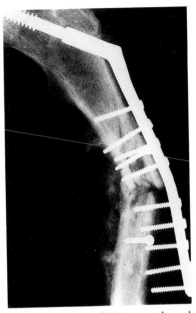

Fig. 4.90 Plate breakage or pulling out of fixation is usually due to poor technique such as leaving a defect opposite the plate.

KEY POINTS

a. **Remove the old plate and screws.**
b. **Reapply a plate that is four holes longer than the broken one. If the screws were tight in the old plate then the same screw holes can be used (provided the reduction is satisfactory).**
c. **Pack a generous amount of cancellous bone around the fracture site. This bone is best obtained from the inner table of the patient's iliac crest on the same side.**
d. **Do not allow weight bearing for six weeks and then it should be graduated weight bearing provided the radiographs show that the graft is consolidating.**

5. Cast bracing

Fractures of the femur in some centres are treated by cast bracing after initial reduction and traction. This is not a popular method of treatment for the following reasons.

1. The technique requires some expertise in application of the cast brace which must be well fitting (Fig. 4.93), and in particular the knee hinges must be accurately placed.
2. In most cases some residual deformity (shortening and angulation) results. The more expert you are the less the shortening and angulation.
3. It is unsuitable for fractures in the proximal half of the femur.
4. Shortening and angulation can develop insidiously. Angulation can be corrected by wedging the cast (Fig. 4.94), but some degree of shortening always occurs in fractures that are not in anatomical alignment.

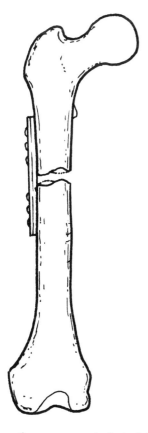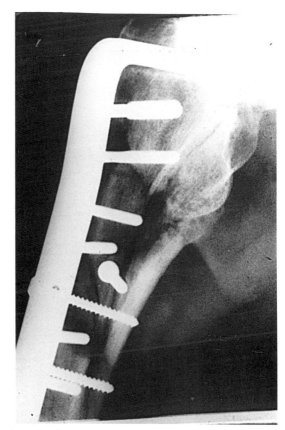

Fig. 4.91 The other common technical fault is to plate the fracture apart.

6. Circlage wiring

This technique of fracture fixation either alone or in combination with intramedullary nailing has its advocates in management of fractures of the femur. Many now believe this technique has been superseded by the advent of locked nails.

Some techniques are shown in Fig. 4.95.

Circlage wires may cause 'ringbarking' of the shaft of the femur by pressure necrosis on the periosteal blood supply. The wires can become embedded in the femur and prove impossible to remove in toto after a few months (Fig. 4.96). As they are only required for short term stability the wires must be removed early (eight to twelve weeks) if the radiographs are satisfactory.

Certainly the stability obtained by circlage wiring is not comparable with other methods of internal fixation.

7. External fixation

The place for external fixation in treatment of fractures of the femur is undoubtedly in severe compound injuries, and in secondary fixation of the infected fracture where other fixation methods have been removed. Probably the simplest system to use is the Wagner leg lengthening apparatus (Fig. 4.97).

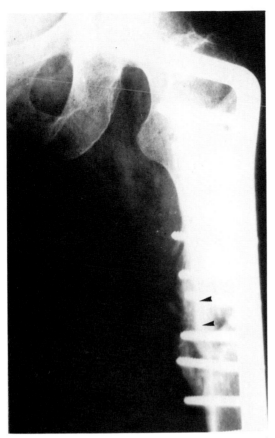

Fig. 4.92 Replating and bone grafting using different screw holes and a longer plate.

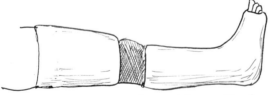

Fig. 4.93 The elements of a cast brace. The leg cast, the thigh cast and the padded knee sock. Yet to be added are the knee hinges.

There are many other external fixation systems in use such as the Hoffman and Orthofix systems.

The blocks of three pins and the triangula-

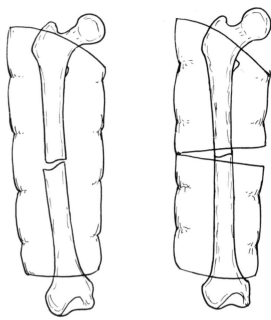

Fig. 4.94 Angulation can be corrected by wedging the thigh cast.

tion techniques of the Hoffman system make it the system I favour (Fig. 4.98).

Problems include:

1. Pin loosening which may require resiting of the pins. Pin tract infection may persist.
2. A tendency to delayed and even non union as the fracture whilst held in alignment is not rigidly held and can even be held apart.

TREATMENT

Wherever possible (from a soft tissue healing point of view) internally fix the fracture and bone graft it at about six weeks.

8. Infection after internal fixation

Deep infection after internal fixation is a serious problem as the fixation can rapidly

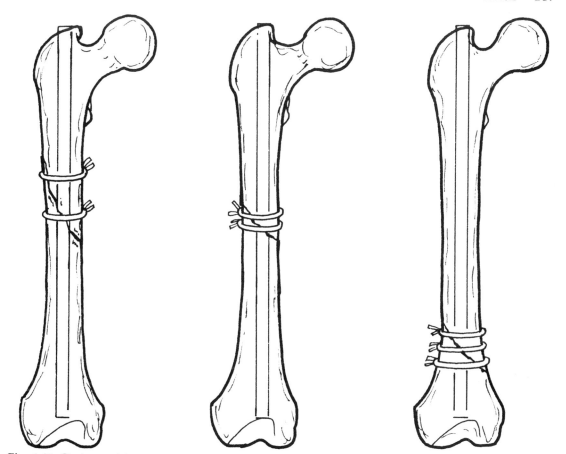

Fig. 4.95 Circlage wiring can be used alone or in conjunction with medullary nailing.

become compromised and loosen resulting in the position being lost. Osteomyelitis may become chronic and present long term problems.

TREATMENT

Superficial wound infection will usually repond to dressings and antibiotics where necessary.

Deep infection requires adequate drainage, antibiotics and on occasions an irrigation system.

LEAVE THE FIXATION IN PLACE IF IT IS PROVIDING STABILITY. Remove the fixation if stability has been lost, and restabilize with either external fixation (Fig. 4.98) or in a plaster cast. Stability can be tested clinically by stressing the fracture to see if there is mobility. The radiograph may show loosening of the screws and movement of the plate.

Remove any obviously dead bone and necrotic tissue.

Rarely will one see a plate on view

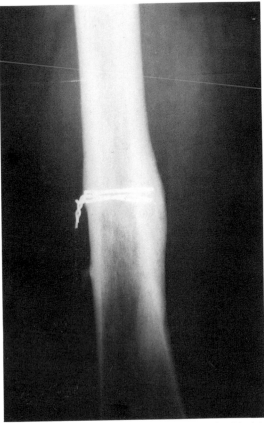

Fig. 4.96 Circlage wires can become embedded in the bone and prove impossible to remove.

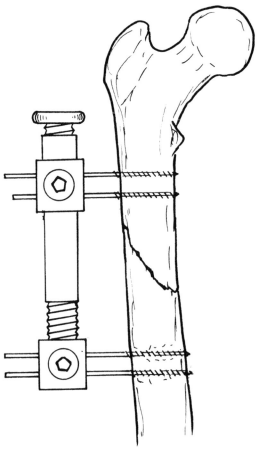

Fig. 4.97 The Wagner leg lengthening apparatus can be used as an external fixateur.

after internal fixation of a fracture of the femur as the soft tissue cover is so much better. If it does occur, it is not a cause for alarm, and does not in itself justify removal of the plate. If possible continue with moist dressings and allow the fracture to unite. Then skin coverage and wound healing are relatively easily obtained.

If you remove a plate on view before the fracture is united you convert a stable ununited fracture without wound healing into an unstable infected fracture. It is a different matter if the fixation is loose. In this case the loose fixation must be removed and the fracture restabilized.

(vi) Refracture of the shaft

This is a rare complication provided the internal fixation is allowed to stay until the fracture has fully consolidated. In cases

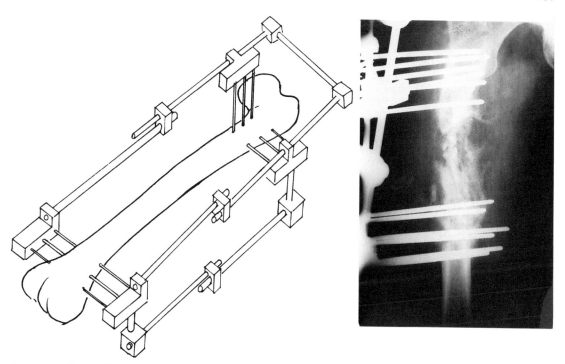

Fig. 4.98 The Hoffman system can be used in two planes and locked together to triangulate the fixation.

treated by medullary nailing the nail should stay in place for about 18 months and the radiograph should show convincing evidence of consolidation before the nail is removed (Fig. 4.99).

TREATMENT

Refractures tend to be undisplaced and are relatively easily internally fixed and bone grafted.

(vii) Nerve and vascular injuries

While it is always possible to have nerve and vascular injuries in any compound fracture, these are rare in fractures of the femur. Damage can occur to the femoral artery or vein during open reduction and fixation. A more common finding is damage to one of the circumflex branches of the profunda femoris artery which encircle the femur (Fig. 4.100).

In these cases the most common method of damage is to lacerate the artery and vein whilst drilling a hole in the femur and this can lead to immediate haemorrhage or result in the formation of an arterio-venous fistula. If this is large enough it can cause cardiac failure. A bruit can be heard over the fistula.

TREATMENT

In all cases of vascular damage the two R's apply: recognize the damage and repair it.

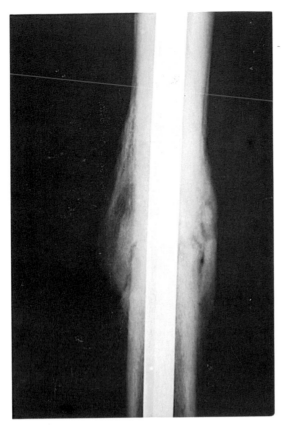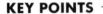

Fig. 4.99 Refracture of the shaft of the femur can occur after removal of the fixation. This nail is not ready for removal.

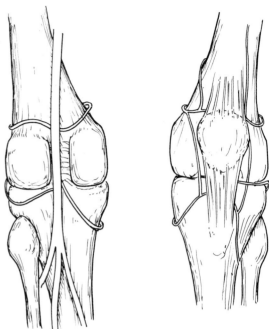

Fig. 4.100 The rich circulation around the femur distally.

KEY POINTS

a. **Unless you are competent at vascular repair and grafting obtain help. Major vessels must be restored within a few hours.**

b. **Major vessel damage requires repair or grafting and internal fixation of the fracture.**

c. **A damaged circumflex branch of the profunda artery can be ligated.**

d. **Suspicion of an arteriovenous aneurysm or a false aneurysm due to partial severing of an artery may be raised by the presence of a pulsating swelling with an audible bruit and can be confirmed by an arteriogram. Ligation of the feeding vessels will suffice for the small vessel lesion, but an aneurysm involving a major vessel will require expert repair.**

The only significant nerve injury that occurs during treatment of fractures of the femur is to the lateral popliteal nerve (peroneal nerve). Improperly applied traction (i.e. skin traction applied above the knee, or prolonged and strong skeletal traction through the tibia) can cause paralysis which may be permanent, resulting in a foot drop. Occasionally paralysis of the anterior compartment muscles comes about from pressure on the nerve over the head the fibula as the leg lies in external rotation against a splint.

TREATMENT

If traction is used, it is essential that the splintage is checked daily to see that there is no pressure over the nerve. Permanent nerve damage will require the provision of a method of dorsiflexion of the foot. This can be carried out with: a toe raising orthosis; a tendon transfer such as the transfer of the tibialis posterior tendon to the dorsum of the foot or a bone block to prevent plantar flexion beyond a certain point.

(viii) Difficult combined injuries

1. Fractured shaft and neck of femur

This combination of fractures in the one femur presents specific problems in recognition and in fixation. The fracture of the neck may be overlooked particularly if it is incomplete initially. Occasionally the fracture of the neck of the femur can follow medullary nailing where the entry point of the nail is placed too far medially (Fig. 4.101). This occurs especially when the retrograde method of inserting the nail from the fracture site is used, together with hammering the nail from below.

TREATMENT

The Zickel nail combines intramedullary nailing with a cross pin in the neck of the femur (Fig. 4.102). I find it difficult to use and get both fractures

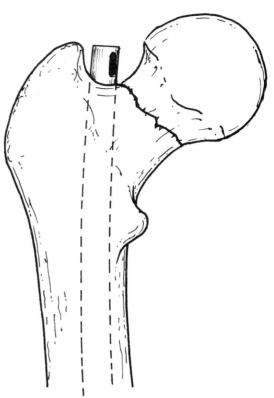

Fig. 4.101 Fracture of the neck of the femur may result from hammering the nail from below and the nail coming out medially in the neck.

aligned and well fixed. I suggest the use of a medullary nail and cross threaded pins or screws for the neck of the femur going around the nail (Fig. 4.103) for fractures down the shaft, use a long angle plate if the fracture of the femoral shaft is in the upper third. The Huckstep nail (Fig. 4.72) can also be used.

2. Fractured femur and dislocated hip

This is the classic trap for the unwary who disobey the axiom that you must see the joint above and below the fracture in examining

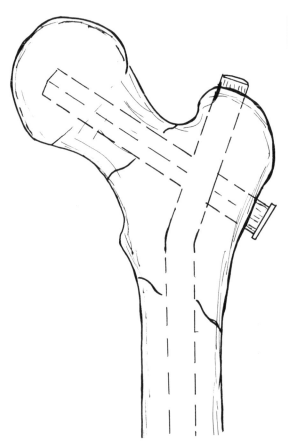

Fig. 4.102 The Zickel nail has a medullary component and a cervical pin that fits through the main nail.

the radiographs of any injury. It is all to easy to assume that all the deformity is due to the fracture of the shaft and a dislocation is not suspected until it is too late to reduce the dislocation by simple means (Fig. 4.104).

TREATMENT

If the dislocation is recognized then the treatment follows standard lines namely:

1. **Reduce the dislocation, if possible by closed reduction, if necessary by open reduction.**

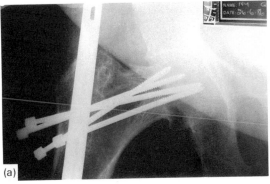

(a)

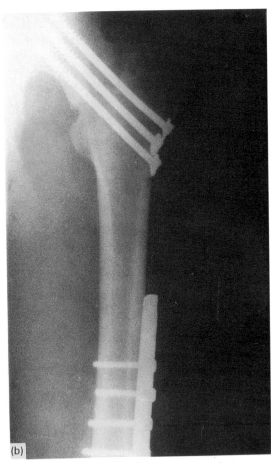

(b)

Fig. 4.103 (a) Knowles pins or compression screws can be inserted around a medullary nail to control a fractured neck of femur, (b) in combination with a fracture of the shaft of the femur.

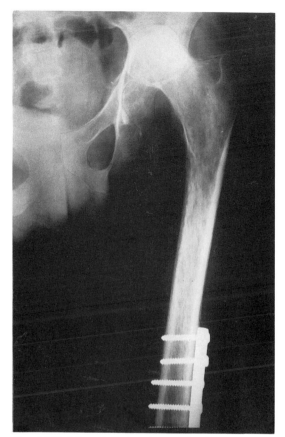

Fig. 4.104 Missed dislocation of the hip joint with a fractured shaft of the femur.

2. Reduce and internally fix the fracture of the femur.
3. Apply simple traction to the leg for three weeks.

If the dislocation is unrecognized for several weeks then open reduction of the hip will be necessary. This procedure is difficult due to the filling in of the acetabular fossa with scar tissue and the dense adhesions that form around the head and neck of the femur.

┌─ **KEY POINTS** ──────────┐

The operation is difficult and bloody. It is best to carry out dissection around the head and the acetabulum on the bone plane.
  Hip movement and function are unlikely to be good if open reduction and extensive dissection are necessary, but any secondary operative measures such as arthrodesis or hip replacement are facilitated by having the hip in place.

└──────────────────────────┘

3. Ipsilateral fractures of femur and tibia

This combination of fractures is virtually impossible to treat successfully (when one or both fractures are displaced) by conservative measures such as plaster and traction. What tends to happen is that the patient ends up with a limb that is short and malrotated. In addition there is commonly loss of knee movement.

TREATMENT

The tibial fracture should be openly reduced and plated or nailed in anatomical alignment. This makes alignment and length easy to judge in the femur which should then be internally fixed by an intramedullary nail or plate and bone graft according to the type and site of the fracture.

┌─ **KEY POINTS** ──────────┐

a. If there are multiple fractures in the tibia (i.e. at the ankle and middle third) then fix the most distal fracture first and this will

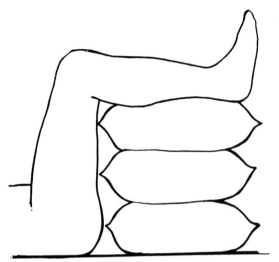

Fig. 4.105 The 90/90 position is a good postoperative position for combined operations on the femur and tibia.

make alignment of the more proximal fracture easier.

b. **The tibial fracture can be fixed under a tourniquet giving a bloodless field and minimizing blood loss. The tourniquet can then be removed and the femur fixed.**

c. **At the conclusion of both operations the leg should be rested initially with the leg elevated and the hip and knee flexed (Fig. 4.105) for a few days and then mobilization of all joints in the lower limb commenced.**

4.1.7 DISTAL THIRD

These fractures present particular problems in achieving and maintaining alignment by conservative means and commonly there is posterior angulation (Fig. 4.106(a)) with subsequent loss of knee function.

Particular problems with these fractures are:

1. Difficulties in controlling posterior angulation, malunion
2. Involvement of the articular surface in the fracture, loss of knee function and traumatic arthritis
3. There is often gross comminution (Fig. 4.106(b)), and it is easy to leave a defect opposite the plate, plate breakage and non union
4. This fracture can be associated with vascular damage to the femoral or popliteal vessels, see above for treatment
5. Loss of knee movement due to quadriceps damage and adhesions

TREATMENT

There is no more satisfying fracture to reconstruct than this one. I believe that the use of the AO 90° angle plate and cross screws together with bone grafts will allow excellent reconstruction of this fracture with the probability of good knee function.

KEY POINTS

a. **It is important to open the knee joint and reconstruct the femoral condyles (where split) first. Use Kirschner wires to hold the fragments in place while they are lag screwed, being careful not to place the screws where they will cause problems during insertion of the plate. Perfect alignment of the condyles is essential (Fig. 4.107).**

b. **Placement of the blade of the plate is important so that it does not go into the knee joint or**

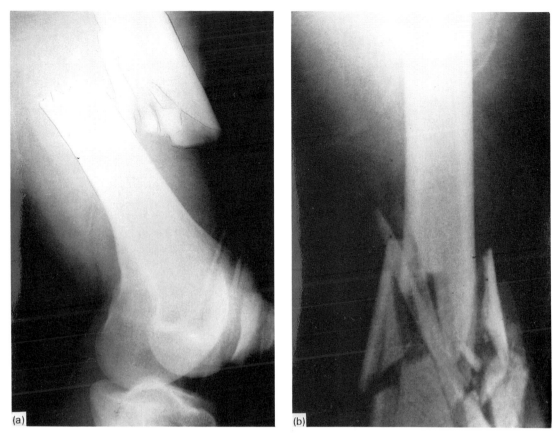

Fig. 4.106 Fractures of the distal third of the shaft of the femur commonly have: (a) posterior displacement and angulation; (b) gross comminution.

even damage the popliteal artery (Fig. 4.108).

c. The angle of insertion of the blade is important as the condylar unit of the fracture must be aligned correctly with the shaft. Remember that on the lateral side of the femur where the plate will lie, the condyles are offset from the shaft and if care is not taken the shaft will be pulled laterally and will not be in its normal relationship with the condyles (**Fig. 4.109**).

d. In comminuted fractures there is almost always a defect in the distal femoral shaft antero-laterally where a large piece of the shaft gets crushed. This defect must be filled in with bone graft and further cancellous graft from the inner aspect of the iliac crest to support the medial border of the femur opposite the plate (**Fig. 4.110**).

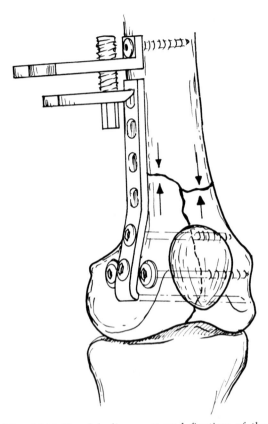

Fig. 4.107 Careful alignment and fixation of the femoral condyles is an essential first step in the fixation of a distal third fracture of the femur.

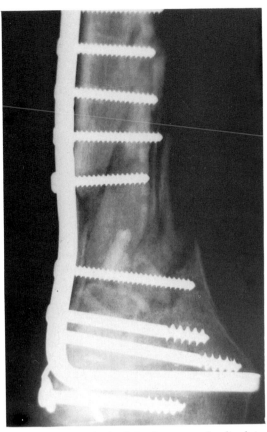

Fig. 4.109 The shaft of the femur can be displaced laterally if the angle of the blade insertion is not correct.

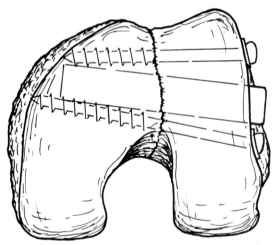

Fig. 4.108 The end on view showing the direction of the blade of the plate that is necessary to avoid penetration of the knee joint.

(i) Malunion

Malunion can be simple angulation or a more complicated combination of angulation and irregularity of the condylar elements of the fracture.

TREATMENT

Simple angulation can be corrected by osteotomy and internal fixation after carefully working out the angular deformity (Fig. 4.111).

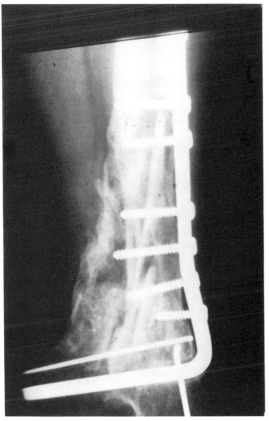

Fig. 4.110 The use of a bone graft is essential in comminuted fractures of the distal third and those that have a defect opposite the plate.

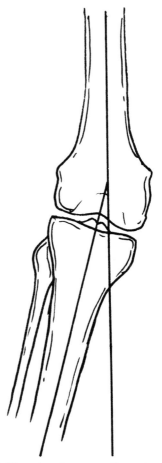

Fig. 4.111 Planning the corrective osteotomy. It is essential to measure the angle of deformity and correction.

KEY POINTS

a. Draw the femoral outline in two planes on graph paper and measure the angle of correction.
b. It will usually be necessary to open a wedge to correct the angulation and not leave any shortening (Fig. 4.112).
c. Insert the blade of the blade plate before you do the osteotomy to facilitate control of the distal fragment.
d. The osteotomy should be in the supracondylar area of the femur as this bone is largely cancellous and will unite quickly. In addition the osteotomy is fully controlled by a 90° condylar blade plate.
e. Remember the femoral (popliteal) vessels are close relations of the femur at this level and can be damaged by a drill or an osteotome. (Urgent vascular repair must be carried out as quickly as possible).

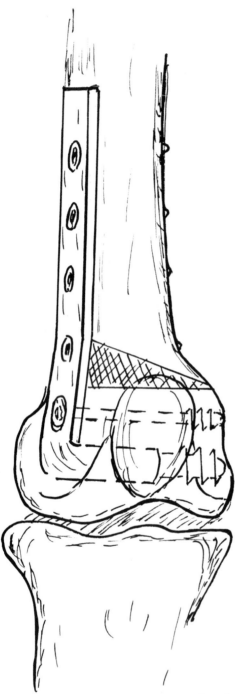

Fig. 4.112 The finished osteotomy with a bone graft and compression plate.

Malunion with gross irregularities of the articular surface cannot be corrected readily and a traumatic arthritis is almost inevitable. This in itself may require resurfacing or other treatment some years later.

The immediate effect of this type of malunion is to give a knee which tends to be stiff and gradually develops increasing pain. In the short term the management will be restricted activity in a work and social sense; weight reduction where applicable and analgesics and anti-inflammatory drugs. In the long term when the patient's lifestyle is being grossly affected by pain and loss of function, the choice will be between an arthrodesis and an arthroplasty. There are very few patients who will accept an arthrodesis.

(ii) Non union

This tends to occur in a small percentage of cases treated conservatively, or in fractures treated by operation and internally fixed with poor technique (Fig. 4.113 (a) and (b)).

TREATMENT

As with all non union the fracture requires:

1. **Correct alignment.**
2. **Secure fixation under compression.**
3. **Bone grafting using cancellous bone to fill in any defects and particularly to buttress the femur opposite the plate.**

(iii) Loss of knee movement

Quadriceps adhesions may follow this fracture or there can be damage to the quadriceps itself. In order to avoid adhesions all operations on the femur and most knee operations should be put on a machine for continuous passive movement (C P M). If this is not

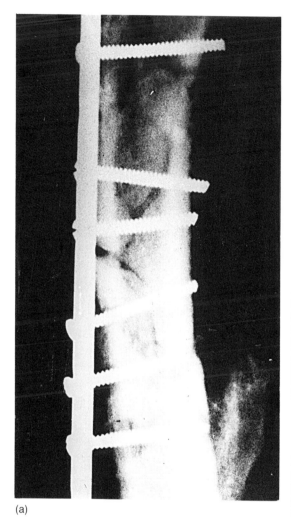

(a)

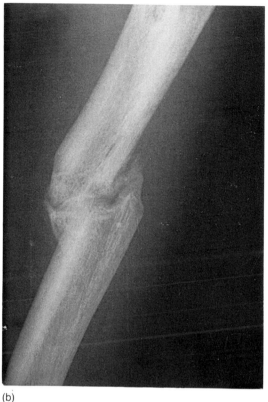

(b)

Fig. 4.113 (a) This fractured femur was internally fixed in a foreign country and the patient flown home. The fixation was poor and fracture became infected; (b) non union of a fractured shaft of the femur treated in traction.

available the knee should be put up in ninety degrees of flexion postoperatively and exercised from this point. Thus if adhesions do occur they will be in the fully stretched quadriceps and not in the shortened muscle when the knee is fully extended.

exercises. A manipulation of the knee under an anaesthetic is worthwhile and may break down intra-articular adhesions. Beware of excess violence during manipulation as you can fracture the femur again.

TREATMENT

When the fracture has united a quad-ricepsplasty can be carried out if no progress has been made with active

---

KEY POINTS

a. In traumatic cases the problem with the quadriceps is almost always due to adhesions of the quadriceps to the femur at the fracture site.

b. **Break down these adhesions, and if they are extensive insert a silastic sheet between the muscle and the bone.**

c. **Drain the wound and use a CPM machine. Be careful to set the machine to give passive motion of about 30 degrees and set at a slow speed. If continuous passive motion is not available put the knee in about ninety degrees of flexion postoperatively. Start immediate active exercises from the ninety degree position.**

d. **Occasionally it is necessary to manipulate the knee under an anaesthetic to free up adhesions that reform.**

e. **Remove any silastic sheeting used after three months.**

f. **Occasionally the deep muscle is so scarred that it is necessary to excise it and lengthen the quadriceps tendon by a V plasty.**

4.2 PATELLA, TIBIA AND ANKLE

4.2.1 PATELLA

This fracture is common and produces a few complications.

(i) Malunion with disruption of the articular surface, traumatic arthritis

(ii) Non union of the fracture with disruption of the patella mechanism

(iii) Disruption of the fracture and rupture of the quadriceps mechanism in the post operative phase

(i) Malunion

Fractures of the patella are of course intra-articular and as such need accurate reduction and good fixation.

TREATMENT

Tension band wiring is the treatment of choice in all fractures of the patella except grossly comminuted and contaminated compound fractures. In the past, excision of the fractured patella was advised in all comminuted fractures and those present in the over forty five age group. It is now conceded that retention of the patella is desirable and the results are superior. Compound fractures with gross contamination and comminution require patellectomy and repair of the quadriceps mechanism.

KEY POINTS

a. **Use a No. 6 atraumatic sternal wire suture which is on a big curved needle and can easily be passed under the quadriceps muscle and the patella tendon (Fig. 4.114).**

b. **A cross K wire may be needed occasionally (Fig. 4.115).**

Malunion with disruption of the articular surface can occur. If the fracture of the patella is grossly comminuted then some roughness of the articular surface is inevitable (Fig. 4.116). However it is best to gather the fragments together using a tension band technique shown above and thus repairing the extensor mechanism of the knee. Simple transverse fractures of the patella should be able to be reduced and maintained in perfect position so that there is minimal damage to the articular surface.

TREATMENT

Gross crepitus and pain in the knee indicate damage to the articulation between the patella and femur after a fracture of the patella. If the rest of the knee is undamaged (this can be checked arthroscopically) then patellectomy and repair of the extensor mechanism is indicated.

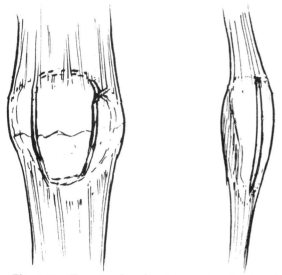

Fig. 4.114 Tension band wiring of a fractured patella. Parallel vertical Kirschner wires can be added.

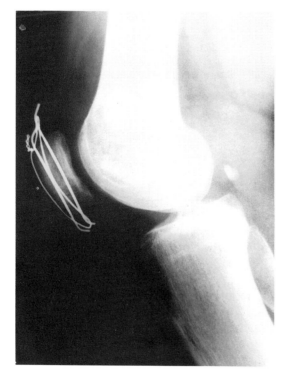

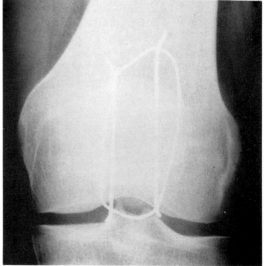

Fig. 4.115 Tension band wiring with Kirschner wires in a fractured patella.

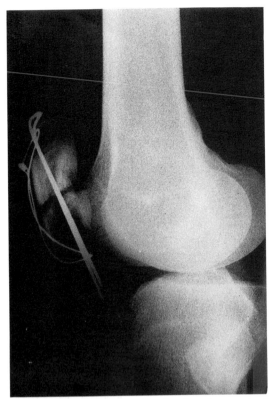

Fig. 4.116 Fractured patella that has been wired. Note the step in the articular surface and the gap at the fracture site. The problem is that the Kirschner wires are not parallel and are too long preventing early mobilization.

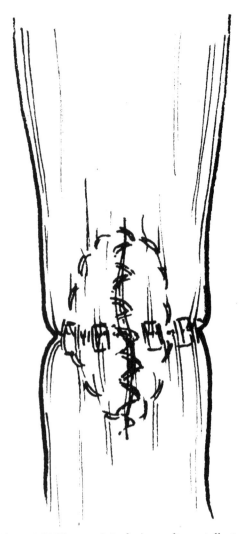

Fig. 4.117 The repair technique after patellectomy. Note the vertical incision in the quadriceps fascia over the patella and the side to side repair. The circular purse string suture improves the appearance of the knee.

KEY POINTS

a. **Where possible the patella should be shelled out subperiosteally and the resultant defect in the extensor mechanism repaired in a side to side manner (Fig. 4.117).**

b. **A circular stitch bunching up the superficial fascia will improve the appearance of the leg when the knee is flexed by giving some prominence over the femur instead of a very flat appearance.**

(ii) Non union of the patella

This is rare but can occur in neglected cases (Fig. 4.118 and Fig. 4.119). What usually happens is that there is spontaneous union in a deformed position or even fibrous union with separation of the major fragments of the patella. The major problem then is that the

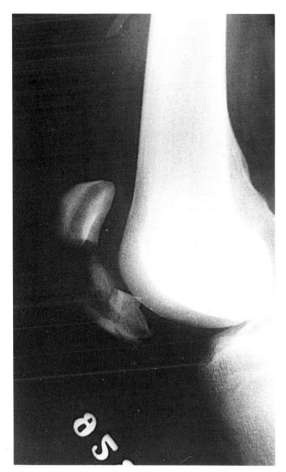

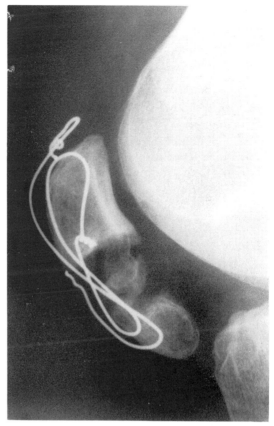

Fig 4.119 This patient went back to full activity before the fracture had united and the fixation failed.

Fig. 4.118 Non union of a patella fracture. The fragments are widely separated.

extensor mechanism is disrupted and even if the patella rejoins by fibrous union then there will be an increase in length of the extensor mechanism and therefore an inability to fully and strongly extend the knee.

An 'extensor lag' creates the following problems:

1. Loss of balance when standing if bumped.
2. Great difficulty in managing stairs or any form of climbing.
3. Inability to run or hurry.

TREATMENT

Reconstruction of the extensor mechanism to eliminate any gap, with tension band wiring of the fracture is the treatment of choice.

(iii) Disruption of the fracture

Disruption of the fracture and rupture of the quadriceps mechanism can occur in the postoperative phase where the fixation is poor or the patient is too active.

TREATMENT

These patients require further operative treatment in the form of a repair of the quadriceps mechanism and tension band wiring of the fracture.

4.2.2 TIBIAL CONDYLES

These are intra-articular fractures and as such need accurate reduction, good fixation and early mobilization to allow full function of the knee.

Complications include:

1. Malunion with poor joint surface, traumatic arthritis
2. Poor knee movement after immobilization

TREATMENT

It is important to understand that there are two basic types of tibial plateau fractures: those that have a cleavage type fracture (Fig. 4.120), and those that have a crushed and depressed segment (Fig. 4.121).

   KEY POINTS

a. **Cleavage type fractures require open reduction and lag screwing in perfect position using long cancellous screws with washers (Fig. 4.122). Closed reduction using traction and compression with an Esmark bandage can sometimes achieve good reduction. Percutaneous screws can then be inserted. It is essential to achieve perfect**

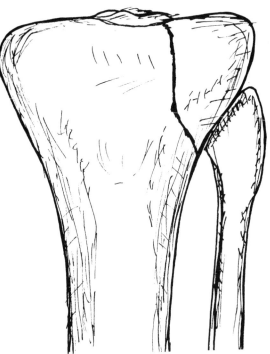

Fig. 4.120 Undisplaced cleavage type fracture of the tibial plateau.

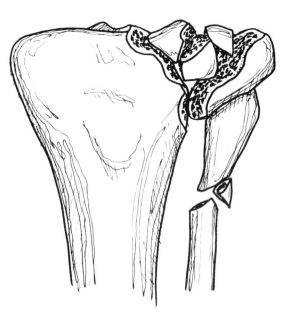

Fig. 4.121 Displaced crush fracture of the tibial plateau.

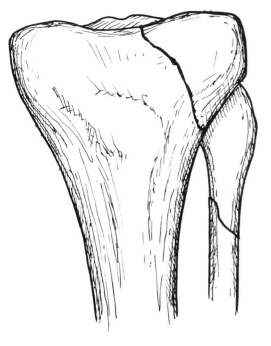
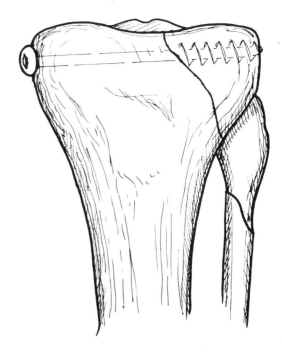

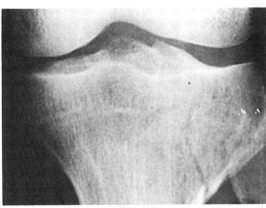

Fig. 4.122 The cleavage type fracture does well with lag screw fixation.

reduction of this intra-articular fracture.

b. Crushed plateau fractures require elevation of the crushed segment with support from below using a bone graft to fill in the defect. The whole area is now stabilized using long cancellous screws and a buttress plate (Fig. 4.123).

c. Mobilization should commence immediately, but weight bearing should be delayed until the area starts to consolidate at about six weeks

d. If a fracture has recently been fixed in poor position then it should be revised.

e. Carry out an osteotomy if correction can be obtained

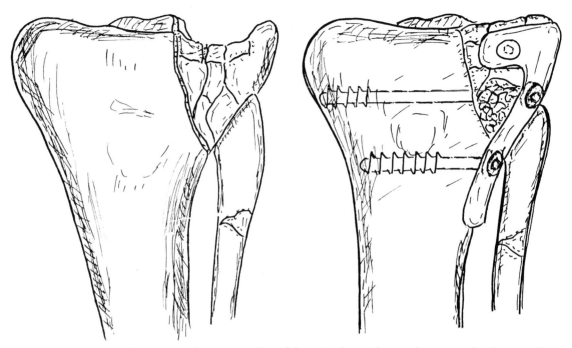

Fig. 4.123 The crush fracture requires restoration of the articular surface and a supporting bone graft as well as lag screws and a buttress plate.

rather than leave an obvious step in the articular surface or an obvious malalignment as seen on the weight bearing radiograph.

Frank traumatic arthritis may require replacement of the affected surfaces with a prosthesis depending on the age of the patient, the weight of the patient (prostheses loosen in overweight patients) and the severity of the symptoms.

Conservative measures such as weight reduction, limitation of activity at work and socially and the use of analgesics and anti-inflammatory drugs will afford some relief for the patient in the early stages of a developing arthritis.

4.2.3 SHAFT OF THE TIBIA

This is a common fracture and has a long list of complications associated with the fracture and type of treatment.

(i) Compound fractures
(ii) Malunion
(iii) Non union
(iv) Vascular and nerve injuries
(v) Overgrowth and valgus after upper third fractures in children
(vi) Complications associated with specific treatment
   1. Plaster immobilization
   2. Plaster incorporating pins
   3. External Fixateur
   4. Medullary nailing
   5. Plating
   6. Cast bracing

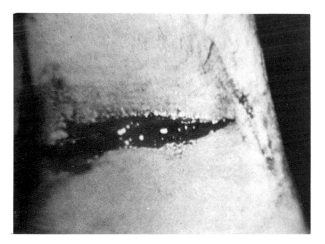 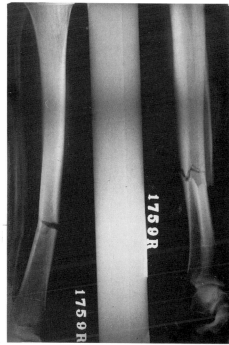

Fig. 4.124 Minor compound fracture of the tibia and fibula (Grade one).

(i) Compound fractures

For practical purposes compound fractures can be divided into three grades of severity depending on the wound, its size and situation; the degree of contamination; and, the mechanism of injury – from within or externally, high or low velocity, cutting or crushing.

The type of bony injury, the type of fracture, joint involvement and comminution, are all important in dealing with the particular problem but do not come into the grading.

Grade 1

These are minor injuries usually being compound because a sharp spike of bone pierces the skin from within (Fig. 4.124). Contamination is usually minimal and the fracture can be treated in which ever way the surgeon chooses including internal fixation.

TREATMENT _____

1. **In the emergency room.**
   a. **Give adequate analgesia after assessing the patient as a whole for other injuries.**
   b. **Apply pressure dressings and elevate the splinted leg.**
   c. **Give anti-tetanus prophylaxis (toxoid booster or TIg 500 i.u. plus toxoid at a different site if not immunized).**
   d. **Take blood for haemaglobin and cross matching and set up an intravenous line.**

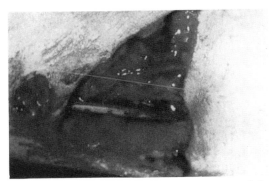

Fig. 4.125 More severe compound fracture of the tibia and fibula (Grade two).

e. **Give a large dose of penicillin intravenously (provided they are not allergic to the drug), say 3 million units. If they are allergic to penicillin give 2 g Keflin.**

2. **In the operating room**
   a. **The wound requires excision of the wound edges after preparation of the leg. Then the soft tissue should be examined cleaned and debrided of dead and damaged tissue (which should be minimal in this grade).**
   b. **Specific treatment for the fracture can now be carried out (such as plating and bone grafting).**
   c. **The wound can be sutured provided there is no tension on the suture line.**
   d. **Antibiotics must be continued until wound healing.**

Grade 2

This type of compound fracture has a larger wound with some soft tissue damage and some minor contamination (Fig. 4.125).

TREATMENT

1. **In the emergency room**
   (a) to (e) as for Grade 1
2. **In the operating room**
   a. **The wound requires excision of crushed wound edges after preparation of the leg. Then the soft tissue should be examined and carefully cleaned using large volumes of sterile water or saline and debrided of dead and damaged tissue.**
   b. **Specific treatment for the fracture may be delayed depending on the amount of soft tissue damage and contamination. If in doubt delay the definitive fracture treatment.**
   c. **Suturing of the wound can also be delayed by two or three days to see that all dead tissue has been removed and that skin closure will not endanger the blood supply to the skin. Loosely pack the wound and apply a plaster cast.**

Grade 3

These are the most severe injuries. They are commonly associated with fractures of the tibia due to motor vehicle and particularly motor bike accidents. There is severe soft tissue (and often bony) injury and the tissue tends to be crushed rather than cut (Fig. 4.126). Contamination with dirt and other foreign bodies is often extreme. The ultimate example of this type of injury is the serious war wound. In these cases it is imperative that a clear treatment protocol be followed as not only is the limb in danger but the patient's life may also be threatened by severe local infection.

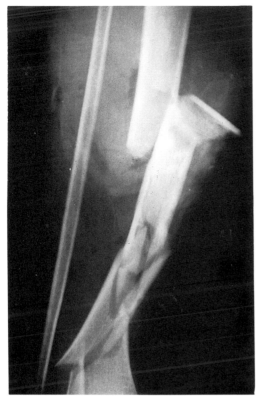
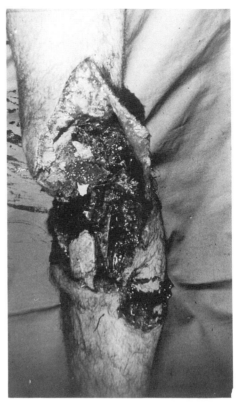

Fig. 4.126 Very severe compound fracture of the tibia and fibula (Grade three).

TREATMENT

1. In the emergency room
   (a) to (e) as in Grade 1
2. In the operating room.
   a. The wound requires excision of the wound edges after preparation of the leg. Then the soft tissue should be examined and carefully cleaned using large volumes of sterile water or saline. A pressure 'pic' is of value but is not essential provided time and care are taken and the wound is thoroughly cleaned ('the solution to pollution is dilution') and debrided of dead and damaged tissue.
   b. Specific treatment for the fracture must be delayed and internal fixation is contraindicated.
   c. Stabilizing the fracture and soft tissues is important. External fixation is the method of choice (Fig. 4.127).
   d. Suturing of the wound must also be delayed by several days and the wound should be simply packed and then inspected under anaesthesia in

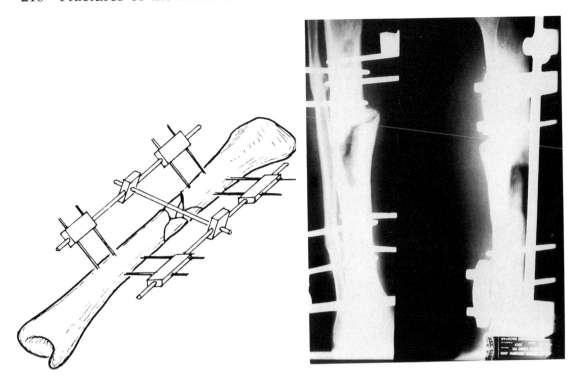

Fig. 4.127 External fixation for a compound fracture of the tibia and fibula.

three days for further debridement if necessary.

e. Delayed primary closure or secondary skin grafting is carried out when the wound is clean and there is no infection.

f. Antibiotics should be given until wound healing and may need to be changed according to the sensitivity of organisms cultured from the wound from time to time.

The key to success in the management of Grade 3 compound fractures is the cleaning and debridement which must be immaculate and repeated third daily until all dead and devitalized tissue has been removed. On rare occasions especially when the blood supply has been compromised and there is gross contamination, amputation may be indicated.

Complications of compound fractures

These mainly revolve around infection and the specific loss of soft tissue in the original damage and subsequent treatment.

They include:

1. Osteomyelitis, usually chronic, can affect the healing of the fracture and give long term discharging sinuses.

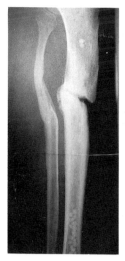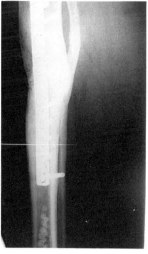

Fig. 4.128 This compound fracture became infected and has now been cleaned out and the soft tissues healed. The fracture was internally fixed and bone grafted and went on to bone union.

TREATMENT

Stability of the fracture must be maintained until union occurs, and any dead or devitalized bone can then be removed. Gaps can be bone grafted even in the presence of a mild chronic discharge provided cancellous grafts are used (Fig. 4.128).

2. Soft tissue problems, mainly skin loss especially over the anterior aspect of the tibia. It is important to obtain skin cover in order to get bone healing.

TREATMENT

Skin flaps, muscle flaps, and even vascularized flaps may need to be used in conjuction with a microsurgeon or a plastic surgeon. Occasionally where all the anterior compartment musculature has been lost tendon transfers may be necessary.

3. Delayed union, is not infrequent especially in Grade 3 compound fractures which are treated by external fixation.

TREATMENT

External fixation should be regarded as a temporary stabilizer for the bone and soft tissues and should be replaced when the wound has healed with internal fixation and bone grafting.

(ii) Malunion

Some degree of malunion is common in many displaced fractures of the tibia treated conservatively by plaster immobilization or by cast bracing. It is a matter of philosophical outlook as to whether you accept shortening, bowing with malalignment of the ankle joint or malrotation and to what degree any of these singly or in combination are acceptable (Fig. 4.129). My personal philosophy is that no shortening greater than 1 cm and no malalignment is acceptable.

TREATMENT

Provided there is adequate skin cover, osteotomy and correction of the malalignment with internal fixation and bone grafting should be undertaken. Bringing the leg out to full length and correcting rotational malalignment is not difficult and gives you very satisfied patients.

┌─── **KEY POINTS** ───

a. **Plan the operation by drawing the radiographs out on graph paper and correct the problem**

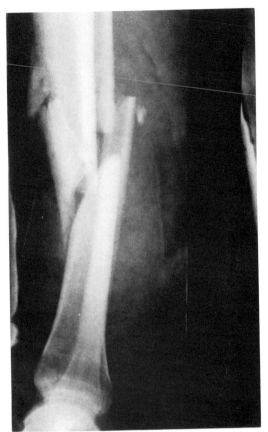

Fig. 4.129 This fracture has posterior and lateral angulation and shortening. I would not accept this position.

d. **Internally fix the fracture/ osteotomy with a plate and screws and if possible lag screw across the osteotomy site; allow for use of four holes each side of the osteotomy site (i.e. a minimum plate size of 8 holes).**
e. **Use a bone graft opposite the plate.**

(iii) Non union

Delayed union and non union of fractures of the tibia are quite common especially in transverse fractures at the junction of the middle and distal thirds which are treated conservatively (Fig. 4.130).

Operative treatment using poor technique which keeps the bone apart can also be responsible for non union (Fig. 4.131).

TREATMENT

Open reduction and internal fixation with a bone graft of cancellous bone from the upper end of the tibia or from the inner table of the iliac crest is the standard treatment for this problem (Fig. 4.132).

(on paper) with scissors and paste.
b. **The osteotomy itself should not be carried out with a saw, but rather with a drill to make several holes along the outline of the osteotomy and then joining up the holes with a sharp osteotome.**
c. **Generally it is better to correct the malalignment at the point at which it occurs and this is usually the fracture site.**

KEY POINTS

a. **Be sure that the fracture is fixed under compression and that there is no defect opposite the plate.**
b. **Use cancellous grafting material liberally.**
c. **If the non union is medially or laterally bowed then the tension side of the bone (the side on which the plate should be placed) is the convex one (Figs 4.133 and 4.134).**

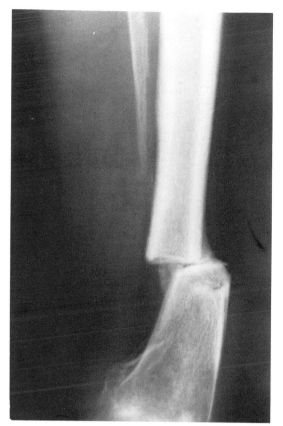

Fig. 4.130 Non union of a transverse fracture of the tibia and fibula at the junction of the middle and distal thirds.

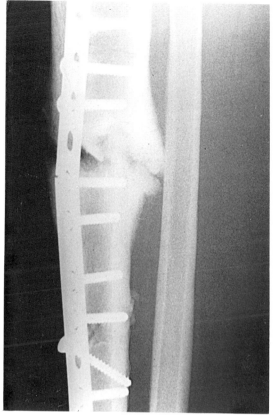

Fig. 4.131 This fracture was plated apart and the inevitably went on to non union and plate breakage.

d. **In some cases where the skin cover is poor medullary nailing and bone grafting is more appropriate (Fig. 4.135).**
e. **Where there is a non union and a continuing open wound it is better to obtain good skin cover first. Often after good skin cover is obtained the fracture will unite quickly.**
f. **Electrical stimulation of bone by internal or external batteries has been fashionable, but at least some of the good clinical results claimed have been due to the improved immobilization provided and bone grafting. I have not found it necessary to use these techniques.**

(iv) Vascular and nerve injuries

Grade 3 compound fractures of the tibia and fibula have the potential to damage the arterial and nerve supply to the limb but seldom do. Damage to the arterial supply occurs mainly in fractures of the upper third

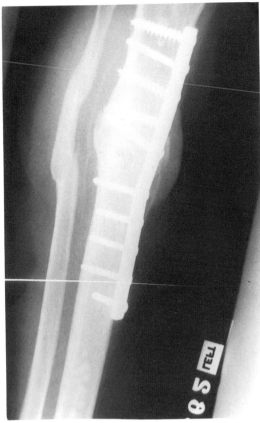

Fig. 4.132 Replating and bone grafting for non union.

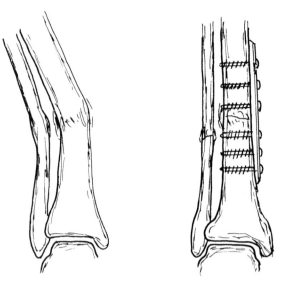

Fig. 4.133 Bowing concave laterally requires osteotomy, plating and bone grafting.

of the tibia as shown in Fig. 4.136. The diagnosis is obvious by the lack of blood supply distally.

TREATMENT

Blood flow must be restored as a matter of urgency by either direct repair or by vein graft. The help of a vascular surgeon should be sought at an early stage. Stabilization of the fracture by internal or external fixation is essential.

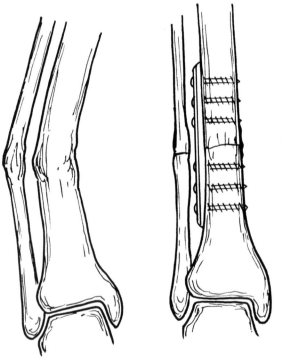

Fig. 4.134 Bowing concave medially requires osteotomy and plating on the lateral surface of the tibia.

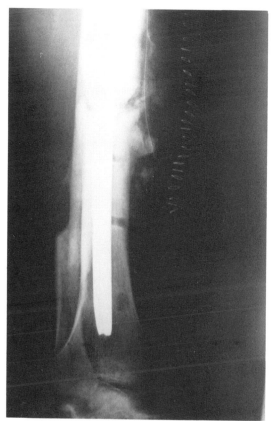

Fig. 4.135 Medullary nailing and bone grafting.

1. Compartment syndromes

This problem is not always associated with a fractured tibia, it can follow heavy exercise. The features commonly seen are:

(a) Severe pain over the muscular compartment involved, rather than over the fracture site. There are three muscular compartments in the leg, each bound by bone and a dense fibrous capsule (Fig. 4.137).
(b) Where there is a fractured tibia involved it tends to be a minor fracture rather than a displaced or compound fracture which would tend to split open the compartments.

(c) Symptoms tend to be delayed by 12–24 hours after the injury or exercise.
(d) What is happening is similar to Volkmann's ischaemia in the forearm. There is swelling in a closed space and initially the venous return is cut off and finally the arterial blood supply (Figs 2.87 and 2.88).
(e) In the leg there is swelling and local tenderness over the muscles involved but the peripheral pulses are almost always present and there is rarely any anaesthesia.
(f) The diagnosis is a clinical one but can be confirmed by manometry.

TREATMENT

Timing of treatment is important as muscle necrosis and fibrosis can occur six to twelve hours from the onset of symptoms. Remove any plaster and carry out a fasciotomy (Fig.4.137 (b)).

KEY POINTS

a. **Fasciotomy should be carried out over all the affected compartments.**
b. **Split the fascia vertically and horizontally. Pack the wound and leave the skin open for a few days.**
c. **Fix the fracture with an external fixateur.**
d. **Neglected cases where muscle necrosis occurs will commonly have a foot drop (anterior compartment) and may need a tendon transfer of the tibialis posterior to the dorsum of the foot (see below).**

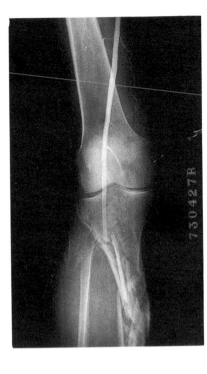

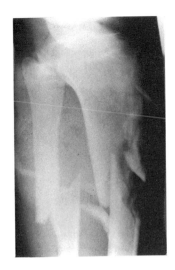

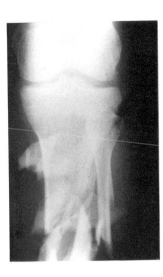

Fig. 4.136 Grossly comminuted fracture of the proximal third of the tibia and fibula with vascular problems.

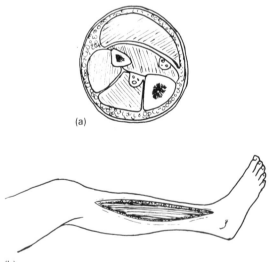

Fig. 4.137 (a) the fascial compartments of the leg seen in cross section. They are bound by dense fascia and bone; (b) the incision for decompression of the anterior compartment. The other compartments are best decompressed by removing a segment of fibula.

2. Nerve injury

Grade 3 compound wounds can be associated with nerve injuries but more commonly the lateral popliteal nerve is damaged by direct injury, traction or pressure as it lies on the neck of the fibula (Fig. 4.138). Pressure over the nerve may cause neuropraxia but it probably only takes six to twelve hours of pressure to permanently damage the nerve and get a permanent foot drop.

TREATMENT

1. **Always pad over the head and neck of the fibula.**
2. **Immediately divide the plaster and pad this area if there are symptoms.**
3. **If palsy and foot drop develop and do not resolve then tendon**

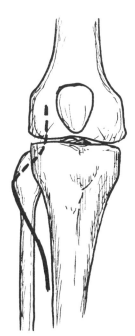

Fig. 4.138 The lateral popliteal nerve (peroneal nerve) is closely applied to the neck of the fibula.

transfer of the tibialis posterior through the interosseous membrane should be carried out.

---

see that the tendon passes freely through the window when pulled down in its new line of pull.
d. **Pass the tendon through a subcutaneous tunnel and insert it either into the peroneus tertius tendon or the cuboid bone. The patient will require plaster for four weeks.**

Reflex sympathetic dystrophy is a rare complication in fractures in the lower limb but can occur and need not be associated with major fractures. The syndrome is characterized by burning pain, swelling, increased sensitivity and sweating.

TREATMENT

This is discussed in the section on Colles' fracture where it is much more common.

(v) Overgrowth and valgus after upper third fractures of the tibia in children

This problem occurs in those fractures caused by a valgus force and deformity and is due to the stimulation to growth caused by infolding of the periosteum (and pes anserinus) into the fracture site (Fig. 4.139(a) and (b)).

TREATMENT

1. **In these fractures open the fracture site and pull out the periosteum and pes anserinus and suture them in their normal place. This prevents the overgrowth.**
2. **Where deformity has occurred (Fig. 4.139 (c)) an osteotomy or**

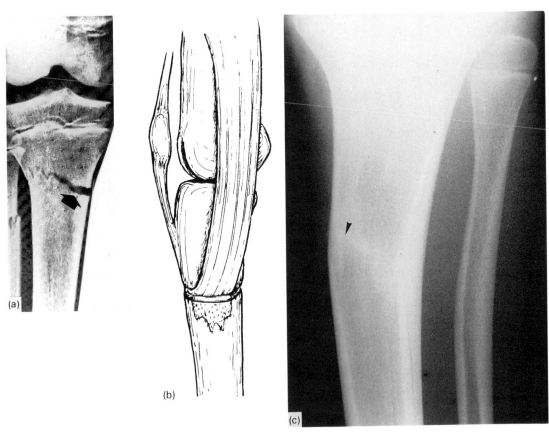

Fig. 4.139 (a) valgus type fracture showing the gap into which the pes anserinus and the periosteum get caught; (b) the pes anserinus and the periosteum in the gap; (c) the varus deformity that results from the fracture in (a) and (b).

osteoclasis may be necessary. One method of doing this is to make multiple drill holes and then break the bone and realign it.

(vi) Complications associated with specific treatment

1. Plaster immobilization

This can give the following problems:
(a) Malunion with shortening and medial bowing.

(b) Delayed and no union in fractures of the middle and distal thirds of the tibia.
(c) Stiffness of the knee and ankle due to prolonged immobilization.
(d) Pressure sores and lateral popliteal nerve lesions when improperly applied.

TREATMENT

These problems and their answers have been discussed above except for (c). Immobilization should be for as short a period as possible and should be followed by a programme

of active exercises, hydrotherapy and graduated weight bearing as soon as the fracture is strong enough. It is important not to wait in a delayed union beyond 20–24 weeks before carrying out internal fixation and bone grafting.

2. Plaster incorporating pins

This treatment can follow the use of an external fixateur or be used in an effort to control the fragments. The problems include:

(a) Holding the fracture apart (Fig. 4.140).
(b) Pin loosening and pin tract infection as the plaster tends to pivot on the pins.

TREATMENT

Pin fixation should be abandoned if the fracture is being held apart or if the pins work loose. If the position cannot be maintained in plaster then internal fixation is indicated after the pin tracks have healed.

3. External fixateur

There is no doubt that the use of external fixation has improved the results in the treatment of the Grade 3 compound injuries. Not only is the bone splinted and aligned, but the soft tissues are also splinted and yet are accessible for dressings. The major problems are:

(a) Occasionally the pin tracks become infected and must be resited.
(b) Whilst the alignment can be well held in external fixation, apposition is generally poor and usually in order to keep the alignment some distraction occurs at the fracture site. Delayed and non union is

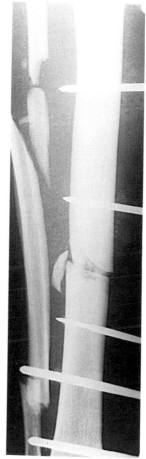

Fig. 4.140 Pins incorporated in a plaster can sometimes hold the fracture apart.

common where external fixation is used as the definitive fixation.

TREATMENT

External fixation through and through the tibia has been superseded by pins put in at an angle so that a triangular frame can be constructed (Fig. 4.141).

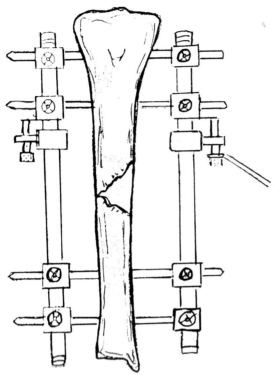

Fig. 4.141 External fixation of the tibia with the through and through method. Triangulation can be achieved with an anterior bar. This method is not recommended.

Use threaded half pins and drill and tap the holes using a jig to accurately locate the sites of the holes. When the acute reason for use of external fixation has passed (i.e. when the soft tissue damage in a compound fracture has healed), change to internal fixation of a suitable type.

4. Medullary nailing

This procedure has never been as popular as medullary nailing of the femur, and is technically more difficult. Some of the problems encountered include:

(a) Penetration of the posterior cortex during insertion of the nail (Fig. 4.142).

TREATMENT

Careful technique will avoid this problem. Re-insert the guide rod and confirm its placement on radiograph.

(b) Bursting the tibia when too large a nail is used or when there is an undetected vertical split in the tibia (Fig. 4.143).

TREATMENT

The choice lies between inserting a small nail and using encircling wires with a bone graft or using a plate and screws (plus bone graft) to hold the fractures. Encircling wires should be removed at six to eight weeks.

(c) Holding the fracture apart
A tight nail can hold the fracture apart and lead to non union. Be sure at operation that you avoid this complication (Fig. 4.144).

TREATMENT

Sometimes the fracture will impact with weight bearing. If it does not then it is best to fill the defect with bone graft.

(d) Nail too long
Penetration of the ankle joint by a nail is due to poor technique and is inexcusable (Fig. 4.145).

TREATMENT

Remove the nail and use a shorter one. The nail should end 1cm above the ankle joint.

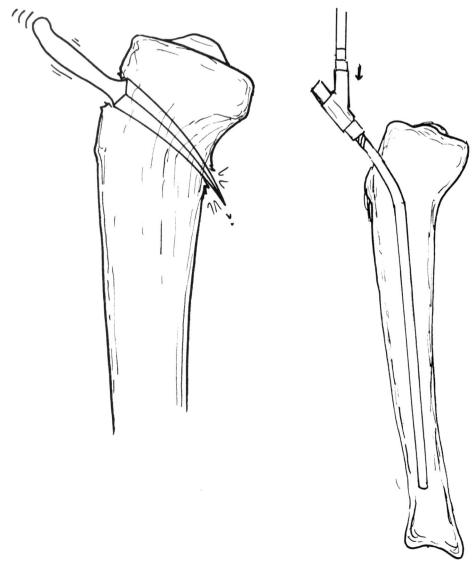

Fig. 4.142 Penetration of the posterior cortex during medullary nailing of the tibia.

(e) Failure to stabilize the fracture in rotation
Tibial medullary nailing does not control rotation well. Locking the nail with two cross screws is important where there is not good rotary control as failure to control rotation will lead to delayed and non union.

5. Plating

This is the most common form of internal fixation and requires an understanding of the biomechanics of internal fixation if the common problems are to be avoided. These include:

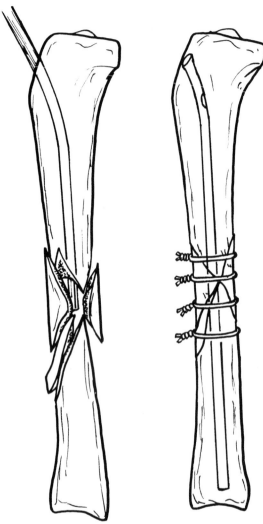

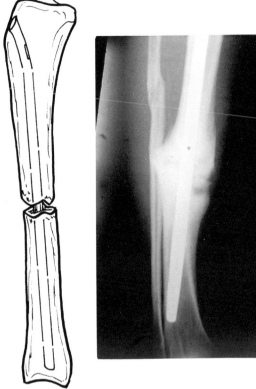

Fig. 4.144 A tight nail can hold the fracture ends apart.

Fig. 4.143 Bursting the tibia is usually due to too large a nail being used or an unsuspected vertical crack. A thin nail and circlage wiring may restore stability with plaster added for external support.

(a) Putting the plate on the wrong side of the tibia The medial side of the tibia is the tension band side and the lateral side should only be used when there is a non union with bowing convex laterally (see non union above). Commonly the plate will break or the system will loosen and lead to a non union if

you leave a defect opposite the plate, plate the fracture apart or put a plate under compression on the wrong side of the tibia (Fig. 4.146).

TREATMENT

Replate the fracture and use a bone graft. The plate will of course be placed on the tension band side of the tibia, the medial side.

(b) Plating the fracture apart, non union, plate breakage This complication is again due to faulty technique. It must be realized that the bone is like a column and the column

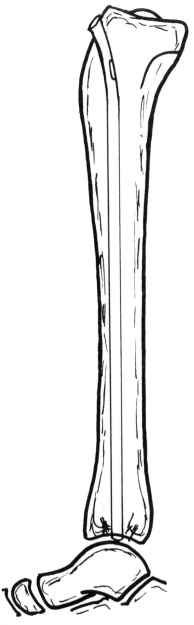

Fig. 4.145 Penetration of the ankle joint by a nail that is too long.

must be restored and compressed together. Leaving a gap or a defect opposite the plate will allow cyclical loading of the plate and it will either loosen or break just as a piece of metal that you bend back and forth will break in your hands. There is always a race between the bone union occurring and the plate breaking, leaving a gap gives nature a big handicap in the race (Fig 4.147).

(c) Infection after plating   There is relatively poor soft tissue cover over the tibia and from time to time we see breakdown over a plate. This problem of a plate on view is not a disastrous one provided the plate is maintaining stability (Fig. 4.148).

TREATMENT

Daily dressings should keep the wound clean until the fracture has united. At that stage the plate can be removed and the wound should heal. Beware of the temptation to remove the plate too soon as you will then have a potentially infected unstable fracture.

(d) Plating and non union   In the past, before compression techniques were widely and correctly used, non union was reported in as many as 30% of fractures undergoing internal fixation. Mostly the problem was poor fixation or leaving gaps. The non union rate in my practice is negligible, but I tend to very frequently support the plate with a bone graft primarily.

TREATMENT

See the section on non union. Replate the fracture if stability has been lost and bone graft the fracture site with cancellous bone from the upper end of the tibia (Fig. 4.149)

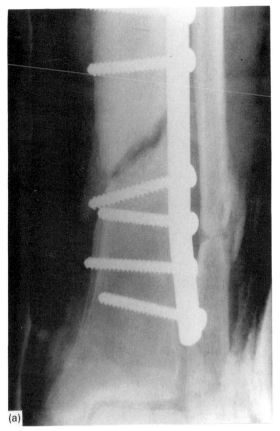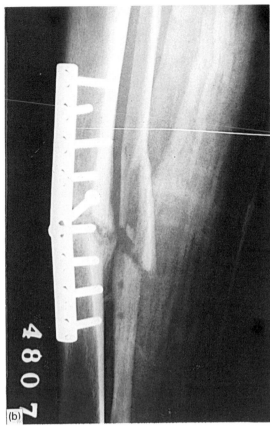

Fig. 4.146 (a) this plate is on the lateral side of the tibia and is holding the fracture apart; (b) defect opposite the plate will often lead to plate breakage.

6. Cast Bracing

The attraction of early return of function with weight bearing has led to the popularity of this method of treatment. It is demanding and requires careful application of a well fitting cast (Fig. 4.150).

The problems include:

(a) Shortening at the fracture site, some degree of shortening is almost inevitable this method of treatment.
(b) Malunion is rare as is non union, provided the cast brace is not applied too soon after the fracture. A period of six weeks in a long leg cast is a necessary preliminary to cast bracing.
(c) Pressure sores under the cast.

TREATMENT

Cast bracing must be carried out correctly or not at all. A properly fitting well padded cast applied after six weeks should avoid the problems. Shortening, angulation and pressure problems may cause you to abandon this treatment in favour of alternative methods.

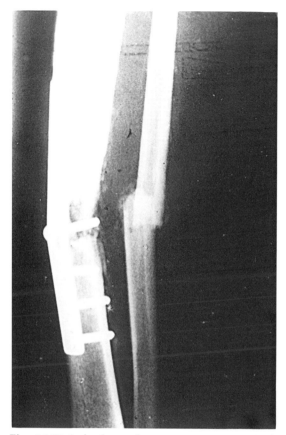

Fig. 4.147 A broken plate means an ununited fracture.

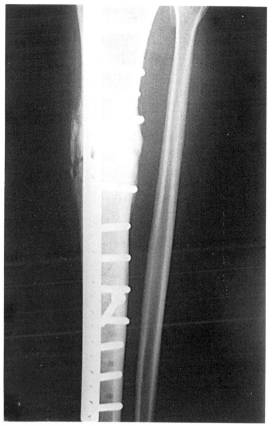

Fig. 4.149 Replating with a longer plate and bone grafting for a broken plate and non union.

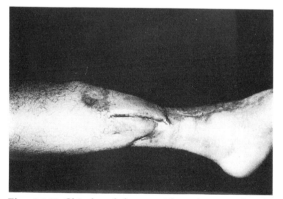

Fig. 4.148 Skin breakdown with a plate on view is not a disaster provided infection does not supervene and stability is maintained. Leave the plate in situ until union occurs.

4.2.4 ANKLE

Displaced fractures of the ankle joint are still a potential source of complications unless reduction and fixation are sound and mobilization is vigorous. Weber's classification and treatment protocol give consistently excellent results.

(a) Type A

There is a fracture at or below the level of the ankle joint of the lateral malleolus, and this may be combined with a vertical split of the medial malleolus. The talus stays with the

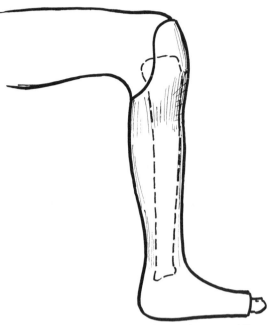

Fig. 4.150 Cast bracing. Note the moulding around the upper end of the tibia.

fractured lateral and medial malleoli (Fig. 4.151).

TREATMENT

As this is an intra-articular fracture accurate reduction is essential. Closed reduction may be successful but I favour open reduction and internal fixation with early mobilization of the fracture.

┌─ **KEY POINTS** ─

a. **Medial and lateral incisions are needed.**
b. **Usually it is best to fix the medial malleolus first in these cases but make sure that the lateral malleolus can be fully**

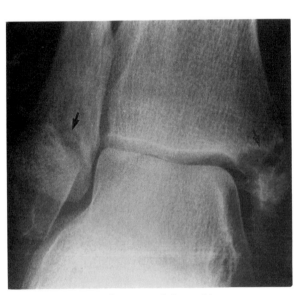

Fig. 4.151 Type A fracture of the ankle.

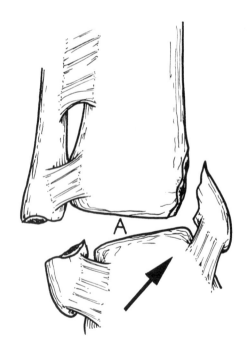

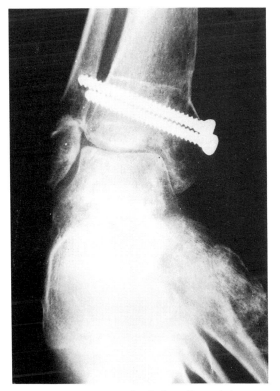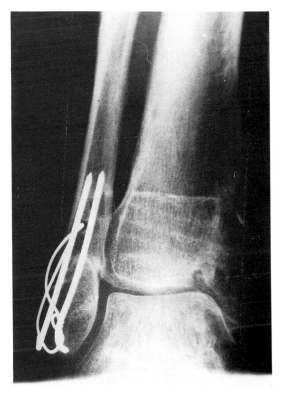

Fig. 4.152 Fixation methods for a Type A fracture. The medial side only was fixed initially causing a non union of the fibula. This was treated by grafting and tension band wiring.

reduced before fixing the medial side.

c. **The lateral malleolus requires either a lag screw, a small plate and screws or a tension band wiring, whilst the medial malleolus may only require two malleolar screws (Fig. 4.152).**

(b) Type B

There is a fracture of the lateral malleolus at the level of the ankle joint extending proximally in a spiral. The anterior tibio-fibular ligament is often ruptured but the posterior part of this syndesmotic ligament is intact so that there is no spreading of the tibia and fibula (Fig. 4.153). There is usually either a rupture of the medial ligament or a fracture of the medial malleolus which is horizontal.

TREATMENT

Closed reduction may be successful, but the position in plaster needs to be checked immediately after reduction and ten days later. Again I favour open reduction and internal fixation followed by early mobilization.

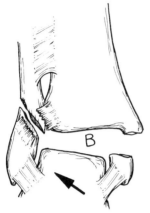 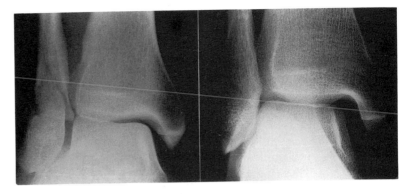

Fig. 4.153 Type B ankle fracture.

KEY POINTS

a. **Reduce the fibula fracture first and when the reduction is complete, plate and if possible lag a screw across the fracture site (Fig. 4.154).**
b. **Now repair the medial side. If a fragment has been detached it is usually a small one and the best way to hold it is with tension band wiring or a lag screw.**
c. **If the medial problem is a ruptured medial ligament then repair it (Fig. 4.155).**

(c) Type C

In this fracture there is a complete rupture of the syndesmotic ligament with a fracture of the shaft of the fibula with displacement of the talus into the space that is opened up between the tibia and fibula (Fig. 4.156). On the medial side there can be an avulsion fracture of the medial malleolus or a rupture of the medial ligament.

TREATMENT

Once again I am in favour of surgical reconstruction of these ankles although closed reduction and plaster fixation can be carried out.

KEY POINTS

a. **Reduce the fracture and stabilize the fibula fracture with a plate and screws.**
b. **Stabilize the tibio–fibular syndesmosis with a non-lag screw (Fig. 4.157) so that these bones are not compressed together but held slightly apart as normally. Compressing them together will prevent the talus from moving in the ankle mortise.**
c. **Remember that the fibula lies postero- laterally to the tibia and so the transfixion screw must be angled anteriorly from the fibula to pass into the tibia.**
d. **Repair the syndesmotic ligament if possible, sometimes**

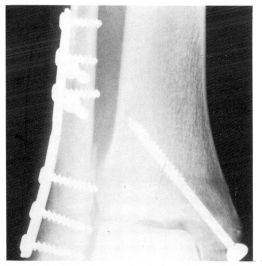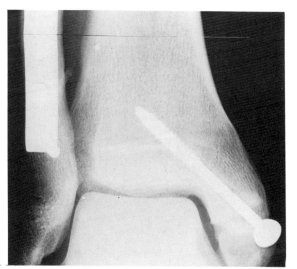

Fig. 4.154 Fixation methods for a Type B fracture.

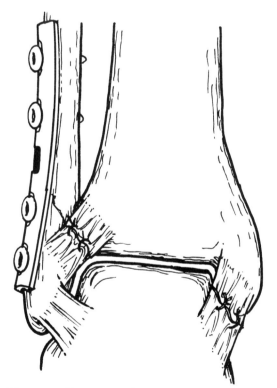

Fig. 4.155 Fixation methods of a Type B fracture.

there is an avulsed piece of
bone to be screwed back.
e. Repair the medial fracture or
ligament rupture.

(d) Pilon fractures

There is no more difficult fracture to treat
than this one as there is so much disruption
of the joint and crushing of the cancellous
distal end of the tibia that it is often similar to
rebuilding a crushed matchbox (Fig. 4.158).

TREATMENT

**Open reduction is essential if a severe
traumatic arthritis is to be avoided.**

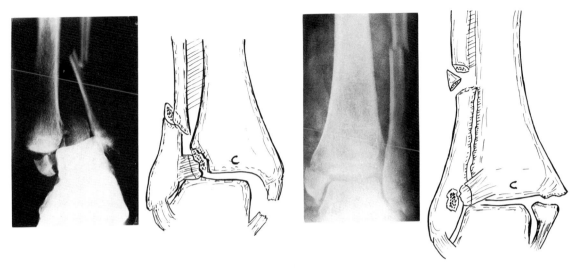

Fig. 4.156 Type C ankle fracture.

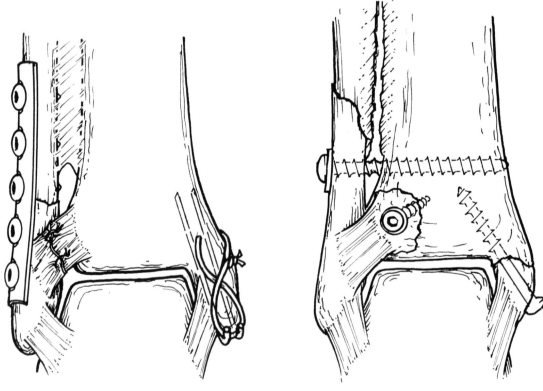

Fig. 4.157 Repair of a Type C fracture.

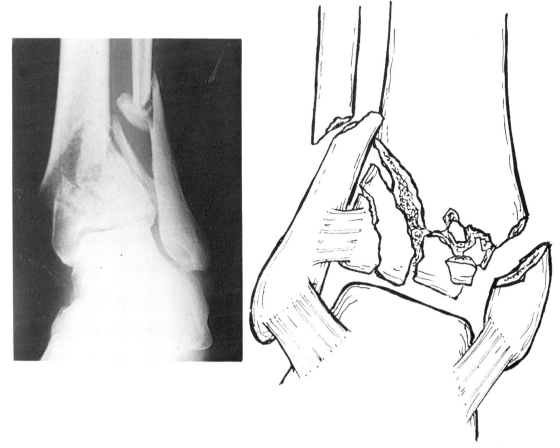

Fig. 4.158 Pilon fracture.

┌─ **KEY POINTS** ────────────┐

a. **Use two incisions so that the articular surfaces can be seen anteriorly and the fibula reconstructed laterally.**

b. **The articular surface can then be reconstructed (Fig. 4.159).**

c. **The defect in the distal tibia will need to filled in with a bone graft.**

d. **Plate the medial border of the tibia.**

└────────────────────────────┘

Complications include:

Malunion

This problem is not uncommon especially in fractures treated in plaster or those cases treated by operation using faulty technique.
  There can be:

(a) Talar shift (Fig. 4.160) where the articular space is not even on all sides. This is usually due to displacement of the lateral malleolus. Displacement of 2–3 mm usually results in some arthritic changes after five years.

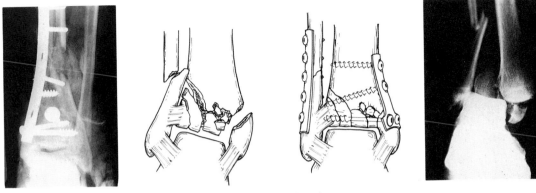

Fig. 4.159 Reconstruction and internal fixation of a Pilon fracture.

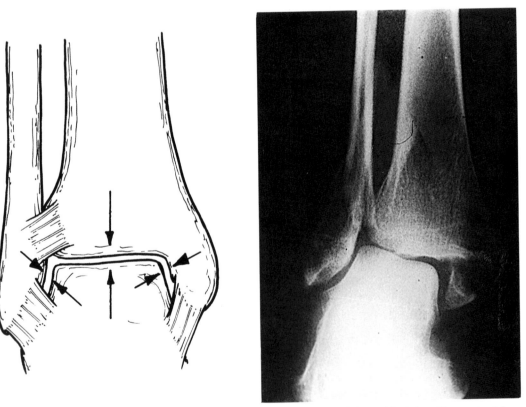

Fig. 4.160 Talar shift allows an increased space on the medial side of the ankle joint. There must be a ruptured medial ligament and the fibula fracture is not fully reduced.

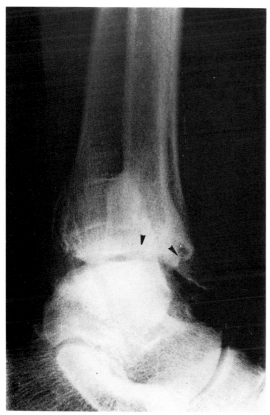

Fig. 4.161 Lateral view of a fractured ankle showing a step in the articular surface and a bony spur anteriorly.

(b) A step in the articular surface (Fig. 4.161).
(c) Fibula shortening with consequent impingement of a wider portion of the fibula on the talus (Fig. 4.162).

TREATMENT

Malunion will cause stiffness and loss of agility. It must be prevented by:

1. **Accurate reduction either by closed or open methods. If you are unable to obtain good position by closed reduction then**
open reduction is essential. At open reduction perfect position must be obtained.
2. **Good fixation is imperative. Closed reduction must be held by a moulded plaster (Fig. 4.163) and the reduction checked on radiograph immediately and then in ten days.**
3. **If the fracture has slipped further closed reduction must be carried out successfully otherwise open reduction is indicated.**
4. **Open reduction must be combined with correct fixation (Fig. 4.164).**
5. **Established malunion may warrant unpicking the fracture and restoring the normal anatomy, especially in relation to restoring the joint surface and fibula length.**

Non union

Delayed and non union can occur in ankle fractures of all types, but is not common. Perhaps the most common type of ankle fracture that goes on to non union is the displaced fracture of the medial malleolus at or below the level of the ankle joint (Fig. 4.165).

TREATMENT

Internal fixation with bone grafting is indicated for delayed and non union (Fig. 4.166).

Post-traumatic stiffness

This is a common complication of ankle fractures especially those that are treated by plaster immobilization and where the patient is reluctant to exercise the ankle. One of the great advantages of good internal fixation is

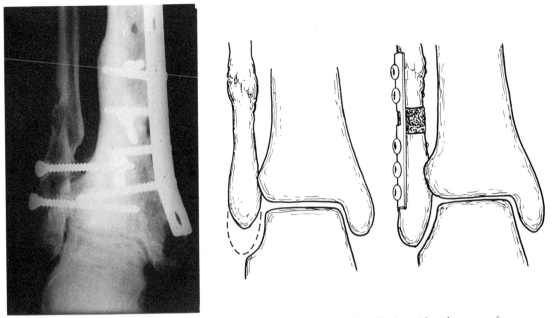

Fig. 4.162 Fibula shortening will allow impingement. Lengthen the fibula with a bone graft.

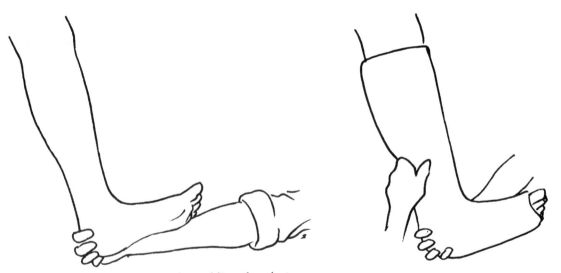

Fig. 4.163 Closed reduction and moulding the plaster.

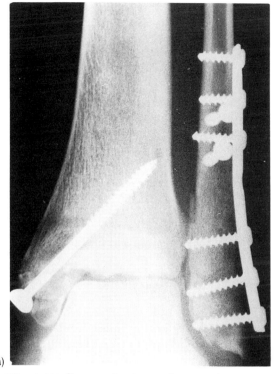

(a)

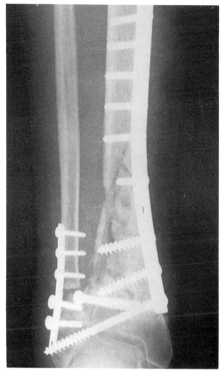

(b)

Fig. 4.164 Open reduction with (a) perfect fixation and (b) poor fixation. Note the tilting of the articular surface of the ankle.

early mobilization of the fracture and return of function of the limb.

TREATMENT

1. **Avoid prolonged immobilization in plaster.**
2. **After plaster immobilization has been removed, or postoperatively in open reduction, a programme of support and elevation together with graduated weight bearing must be carefully followed.**
3. **Rarely stiffness may warrant manipulation under an anaesthe-** tic if no progress is made after prolonged physiotherapy, provided the fracture is firmly united.
4. **Inversion and eversion is the movement that is commonly lost at both the ankle and more particularly at the subtaloid joint. Difficulty in going over rough ground can be helped by the wearing of boots rather than shoes.**

Post-traumatic arthritis

The incidence of this complication has been put at 20– 40%. It is of course more common where reduction has not been perfect.

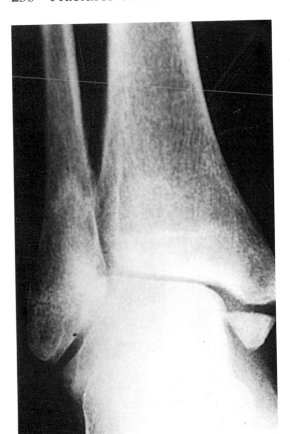

Fig. 4.165 An ununited fracture of the medial malleolus. This needed bone grafting and tension band wiring.

The patients complain of stiffness and difficulty in moving in the morning; aching pain in bad or changeable weather; and pain with activity.

TREATMENT _____

Most patients manage with:

  (i) **Reduced activity**
 (ii) **Weight reduction**
(iii) **Analgesics**
(iv) **Anti-inflammatory drugs**
 (v) **Supportive footware (boots)**

When symptoms are severe enough to significantly alter the patient's lifestyle then arthrodesis of the ankle is indicated.

┌─ **KEY POINTS** ─────────

  a. **There are many ways to arthrodese an ankle (Fig. 4.167).**
  b. **The operation should leave the ankle at 90 degrees in men and in women the degree of plantar flexion should be tailored to any desire to wear high heel shoes.**
  c. **The technique I favour is shown in Fig. 4.168. This application of double compression plates is not difficult and allows early mobilization and weight bearing as plaster casting is not necessary.**
  d. **Be careful not to put the foot in inversion or eversion.**

4.3 TALUS, OS CALCIS AND FOOT

4.3.1 TALUS

(a) Fractures

These fractures are rare but often cause problems. Amongst the complications are:

   (i) Failure to recognize the fracture
  (ii) Failure to recognize the dorsal displacement
 (iii) Fracture dislocations
 (iv) Avascular necrosis
  (v) Delayed union and non–union
 (vi) Malunion
(vii) Arthritis of ankle and subtaloid joint

(i) Failure to recognize the fracture.

Always look carefully at the talus in patients who have multiple injuries following high

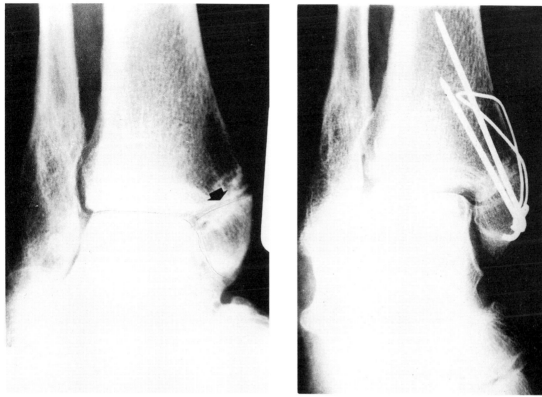

Fig. 4.166 Internal fixation and bone grafting of the medial malleolus is indicated for non-union.

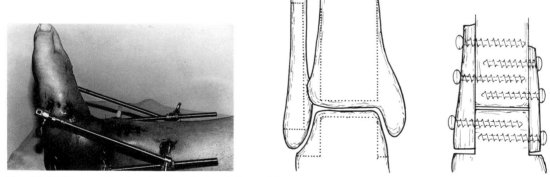

Fig. 4.167 Two methods of arthrodesis of the ankle.

speed automobile crashes especially if they are the driver. The common method of injury is due to forced dorsiflexion of the ankle (Fig. 4.169) against the floor or a pedal in a car.

(ii) Failure to recognize the dorsal displacement

Beware of not recognizing displacement (Fig. 4.170) in this fracture. In both neck and body

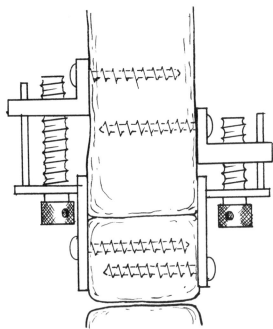

Fig. 4.168 Double compression plates (T-plates) for arthrodesis of the ankle.

fractures the distal fragment is displaced dorsally.

If you favour closed reduction, it must be realized that the talus is only reduced and maintained when the foot is fully plantar flexed. This is not a good position in which to immobilize the ankle, as if a poor range of movement follows, the foot is in the least useful position for walking (Fig. 4.171).

TREATMENT

1. **If a talar fracture is displaced I suggest open reduction and lag screwing with a cancellous screw and washer. The screw should run from anteromedial to posterolateral (Fig. 4.172).**

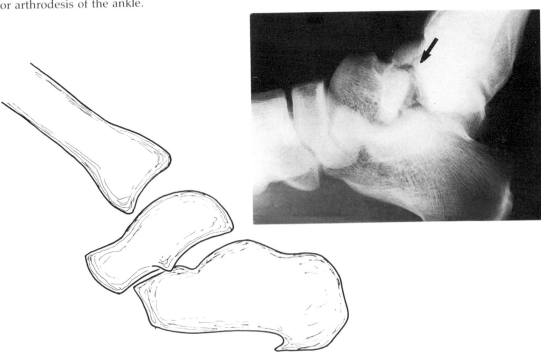

Fig 4.169 Forceful dorsiflexion of the ankle brings the anterior border of the tibia across the talus like a chisel and can cause a fracture of the talus.

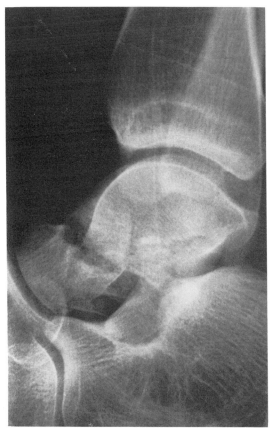

Fig. 4.170 Fracture of the neck of the talus. Note the dorsal displacement of the distal segment of the talus.

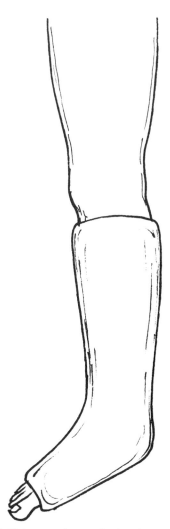

Fig. 4.171 Extreme plantar flexion is necessary to reduce a fractured talus but this is a poor position in which to immobilize a foot as walking will be difficult if any stiffness results.

2. If closed reduction is carried out then plaster immobilization in full equinus and neutral varus should only be maintained for one month and then the ankle should be brought into more dorsiflexion. If the fracture is still unstable at this time then open reduction and lag screwing is indicated.

(iii) Fracture dislocations

You may encounter the following problems:

1. Skin necrosis

When the body of the talus is displaced laterally or posteriorly the skin is stretched to bursting point and necrosis and infection may follow (Fig. 4.173).

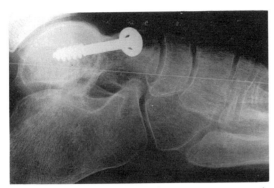

Fig. 4.172 Open reduction and screw fixation of a fractured talus. A cancellous screw and washer should be used.

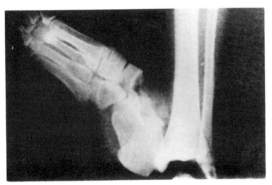

Fig. 4.173 This fracture dislocation must cause skin problems as there is no room for the displaced segment of the talus.

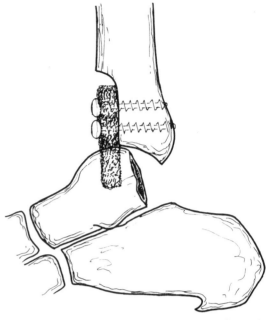

Fig. 4.174 Where the body of the talus is lost it is possible to fuse the tibia to the talar remnant (Blair fusion).

TREATMENT

Immediate reduction of the dislocation is indicated and even some manual traction on the heel in the emergency room after the patient has some intravenous analgesia will often reduce the dislocation (but not the fracture) and take the pressure off the skin.

Necrotic skin must be excised and grafted. Often in these cases the body of the talus becomes avascular and may become infected and act as a sequestrum. In those cases talec- tomy and tibo-calcaneal fusion is indicated (Fig. 4.174).

2. Difficulty with reduction

You may have difficulty with reduction of a fracture dislocation by closed and even open means due to some of the posterior tendons getting caught in the fracture.

TREATMENT

Open reduction will be necessary. Take care not to denude any soft tissue fom the talus as this is important for blood supply. Occasionally the body of the talus falls out on the operating table ... replace it and internally fix the fracture (Fig. 4.172).

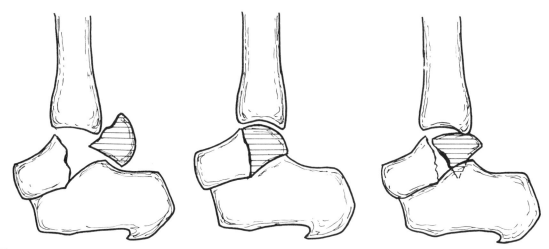

Fig. 4.175 Various types of fractures of the talus with displacement commonly develop avascular necrosis.

3. Avascular necrosis

Most of these fracture dislocations will go on to avascular necrosis (see below).

4. Loss of the body of the talus

In compound fracture dislocations of the talus the body of the talus may be left at the roadside.

TREATMENT

Tibio—talar fusion to the talar remnant gives a reasonably good result (Blair fusion) (Fig. 4.174).

(iv) Avascular necrosis

The incidence of this complication varies according to the type of fracture being 5% in undisplaced and 100% in fracture dislocations (Fig. 4.175). Early and late radiographs are shown in Fig. 4.176.

TREATMENT

1. **Accurate reduction of the fracture or fracture dislocation with internal fixation.**
2. **Protection of the weight bearing surfaces until revascularization occurs. The use of a patellar bearing weight relieving splint is advised (Fig. 4.177).**

(v) Delayed and non union

This fracture is often slow to unite but non union is rare. Fractures that are undisplaced have less chance of disruption of blood supply (Fig. 4.178), whereas displaced fractures often unite slowly and may be complicated by avasular necrosis of the body of the talus.

Fractures of the lateral process and posterior process commonly do not unite by bone unless they are fixed by a screw or wires (Fig. 4.179). Fibrous union is not always painful.

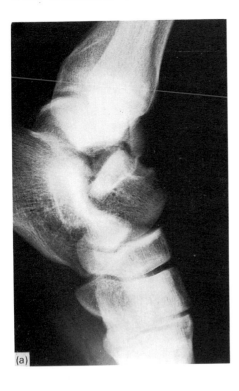

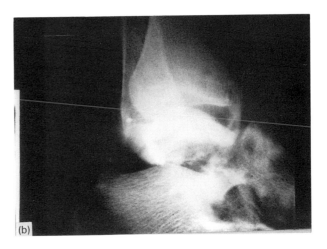

Fig. 4.176 (a) early and (b) late lateral radiographs of avascular necrosis of the body of the talus. Note the collapse of the body in (b).

(vi) Malunion

This tends to occur when dorsal displacement of the fracture is not recognized or when a displaced fracture is put in a cast with the ankle at 90° (Fig. 4.180).

(vii) Arthritis

After comminuted fractures, malunion and sometimes avascular necrosis a frank arthritis can develop. Commonly pain and stiffness in both the ankle and subtaloid joint are present.

TREATMENT

1. **Analgesics, anti-inflammatory drugs, restricted activity and the use of a weight relieving orthosis or even a boot may be of value in the mild case.**

2. **In severe cases where the degree of pain and limitation of activity is severely interfering with the patient's lifestyle an arthrodesis of both the ankle and subtalar joint can be performed.**

KEY POINTS

Put the patient in plaster prior to a fusion, and be sure he or she obtains good relief from simple immobilization and from injection of local anaesthetic into the joints.

(b) Dome fractures of the talus

These are osteochondral fractures that occur when one of the 'corners' of the talus is knocked off (Fig. 4.181). The

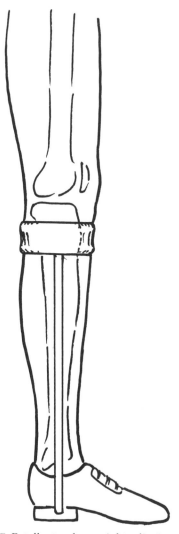

Fig. 4.177 Patellar tendon weight relieving caliper.

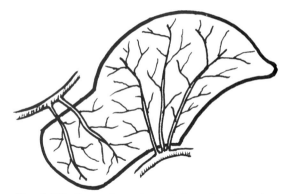

Fig. 4.178 Coronal section of the talus showing how easily the blood supply of the talus can be disrupted by a fracture.

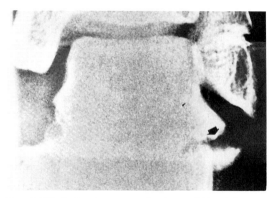

Fig. 4.179 Lateral process fracture of the talus.

condition can be confused with a type of localized avascular necrosis similar to osteochondritis dissecans of the knee.

TREATMENT

1. **Small fragments can be removed by open operation or even arthroscopically.**

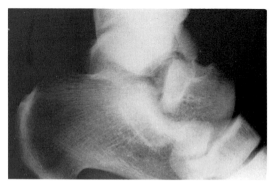

Fig. 4.180 Displacement of a fracture of the body of the talus with the ankle at 90°.

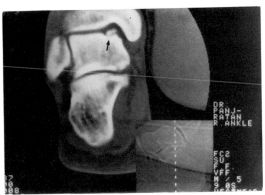

Fig. 4.181 CT scan of an osteochondral fracture of the talus.

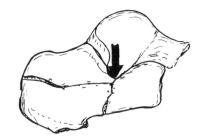

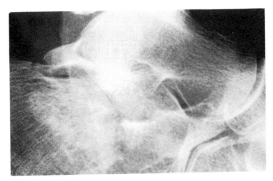

Fig. 4.182 Fracture of the os calcis with distortion of the heel, and a rough bed for the peroneal tendons.

2. **Large osteochondral fragments need to be replaced and held in place with buried pins or Herbert screws (these have a head that can be buried).**
3. **The joint should be protected from weight bearing loads for eight weeks while the fracture and articular surface heal.**

4.3.2 OS CALCIS (CALCANEUM)

This fracture usually occurs in a fall from a height. Displaced fractures involving the subtaloid joint commonly leave disability.

These patients may have:

1. Distortion of the heel; broadening and irregularity (Fig. 4.182).
2. Loss of movement, particularly inversion and eversion.
3. Pain on walking especially over rough ground.
4. Difficulty in finding comfortable footware.
5. Other injuries; a fracture of the other os calcis or a crush fracture of the lumbar spine.

TREATMENT

Controversy still rages over the treatment of depressed fractures of the os calcis where the normal angle is lost in the subtaloid joint. The pessimists say that the damage is complete and the subtaloid joint will not work, whereas the optimists say that restoring the angle and shape of the joint does allow for better function.

If the conservative approach has been taken then you can carry out the following measures:

a. **Lateral prominences can be trimmed. A common source of pain is from the peroneal tendons being caught laterally. This can be seen on a tenogram and occa-**

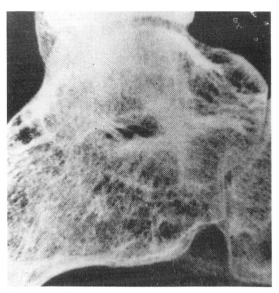

Fig. 4.183 Subtaloid fusion.

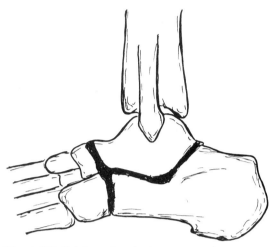

Fig. 4.184 Triple arthrodesis.

sionally a plain radiograph (Fig. 4.182).

b. **Arrange a change in employment, from a job climbing ladders and standing or going over rough ground, to a sedentary job.**

c. **Persistent pain on walking may be helped by a subtaloid fusion (Fig. 4.183). I suggest that you try the patient in a walking plaster first to see if the symptoms are relieved.**

d. **In some case a triple arthrodesis is needed as there is also damage to the calcaneo-cuboid joint (Fig. 4.184).**

e. **Boots that are made to measure often give some relief to the patient's symptoms.**

AFTER OPERATIVE TREATMENT

Persistent pain may be relieved by subtaloid fusion or a triple arthrodesis but a trial of plaster immobilization is suggested as a first step.

4.3.3 CUBOID AND NAVICULAR BONES

These fractures are neither common nor do they present problems in management. The exception seems to be:

1. Very comminuted fractures of the cuboid (Fig. 4.185).
2. Fractures of the navicular bone with displacement or comminution (Fig. 4.186).

Comminuted fractures of the cuboid bone can lead to residual pain in the foot.

TREATMENT

If the pain can be localized to one joint by injecting local anaesthetic into the joint and testing for the relief of pain, then a localized fusion will relieve the symptoms.

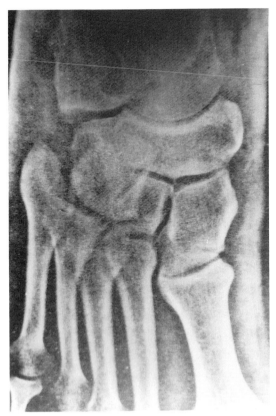

Fig. 4.185 Comminuted fracture of the cuboid bone.

Displaced fractures of the navicular bone can cause localized pain at the talo-navicular joint and also a dorsal prominence that causes problems with footware.

TREATMENT _____

1. **Displaced fractures of the navicular require reduction and internal fixation with wires or a Herbert screw (Fig. 4.187).**
2. **Comminuted fractures that unite with a dorsal lump will require trimming of the lump.**
3. **Pain may warrant a local fusion but only if localized to one joint.**

_____

4.3.4 METATARSAL BONES

(a) Fractures

These fractures are common and present only a few problems. Displaced fratures, especially when multiple, can cause problems with walking. The major problem seems to be when the distal fragment points to the sole of the foot and therefore takes undue pressure during weight bearing. Painful callosities will develop.

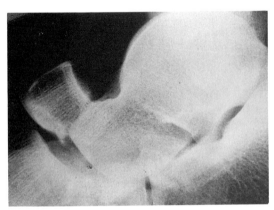
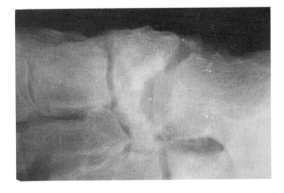

Fig. 4.186 Comminuted crush fracture of the navicular and a displaced segment of the tarsal navicular, the two common types of tarsal navicular fracture.

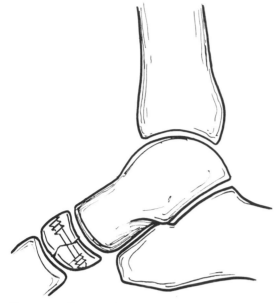

Fig. 4.187 Open reduction and internal fixation of the navicular using a Herbert screw.

KEY POINTS

a. **Use a single dorsal incision centred over the third metatarsal.**

b. **Use a sharp instrument and cut the bone on a slope (distal dorsally to proximal ventrally). Make sure that the bone has been cut completely.**

c. **Ambulation the next day with weight bearing will align the metatarsals for weight bearing and is surprisingly not very painful.**

TREATMENT

1. **Poor position should not be accepted, if necessary carry out open reduction and cross wiring (Fig. 4.188).**
2. **If poor position has developed then corrective osteotomies should be carried out.**

(b) Fracture dislocations

These are serious but rare injuries and present the following problems:

1. Vascular problems, as with displacement the blood supply to the forefoot can be cut off by bony pressure on the vessels or by direct damage to the blood supply where there are compound wounds (Fig. 4.189).
2. Skin problems occur in both compound fractures and in displaced fractures where there can be considerable pressure from

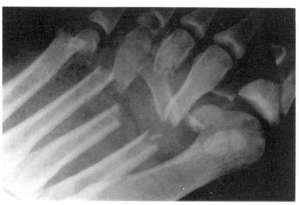
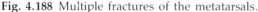
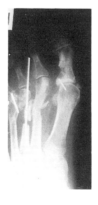
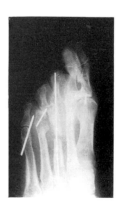

Fig. 4.188 Multiple fractures of the metatarsals.

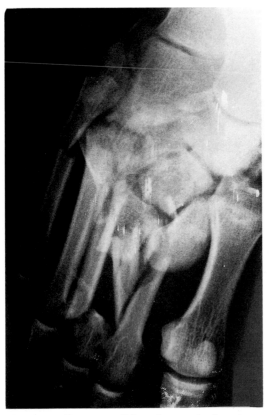

Fig. 4.189 Fracture dislocations of the tarso–metatarsal region such as this are commonly associated with vascular problems.

the displaced bony fragments leading to necrosis of the skin.
3. Failure to reduce and hold the displacement of the metatarsals.

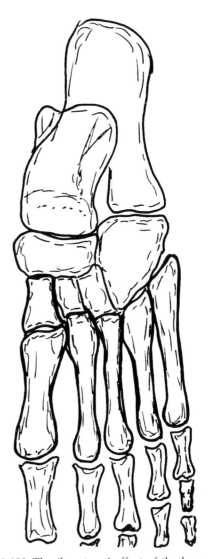

Fig. 4.190 The 'keystone' effect of the base of the second metatarsal which is locked into the second cuneiform.

KEY POINTS

a. **The base of the second metatarsal articulates about one half a centimetre proximally to the other metatarsal bases and locks the metatarsals in place (Fig. 4.190)**

b. **If the second metatarsal base or shaft is disrupted then longitudinal reconstuction** should be carried out using strong Kirschner wires (Fig. 4.191)

c. **Now you can reconstruct the metatarsals and prevent lateral displacement by pinning the other metatarsals to the second metatarsal with oblique wires.**

Fig. 4.191 Restoring the second metatarsal with a longitudinal Kirschner wire to rebuild the 'keystone'.

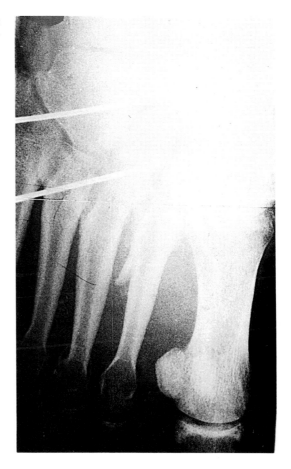

(c) Fractures of the base of the fifth metatarsal

These fractures are common and occur with an inversion injury when the patient 'goes over' on an ankle. The bony fragment is avulsed by the pull of the peroneus brevis tendon.

The problems include:

1. Delayed and non union are not infrequent as there is often a gap at the fracture site (Fig. 4.192).

TREATMENT _____

All fractures with a wide gap will need either

a. Reduction and pinning or screw fixation (Fig. 4.192).
b. Excision of the bony fragment if small and repair of the tendon insertion.

_____

Established non union can be treated the same way. There is one nasty fracture in the fifth metatarsal, a transverse fracture about 1.5 cm from the base. It is often very slow to unite and may go on to non union in spite of the bones being in apposition. This is called the Jones fracture (Fig. 4.193) and responds to bone grafting and internal fixation.

2. Localized tenderness at the fracture site

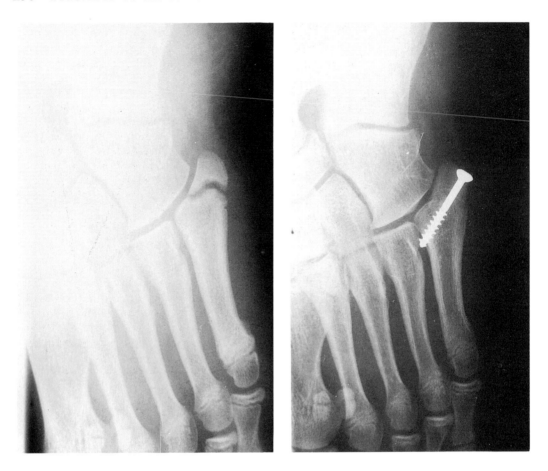

Fig. 4.192 An avulsion fracture of the base of the fifth metatarsal with a gap. This fracture was fixed with a screw.

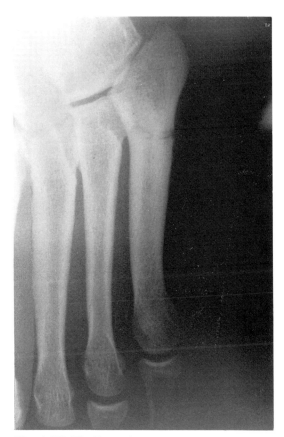

Fig. 4.193 The Jones fracture.

may be due to a prominence that is formed when the bone unites. It may need to be trimmed for cosmetic reasons or to improve comfort whilst wearing shoes.

Femoral fractures

Strathy, G. M. and Johnson, E. W. (1984) Ender's pinning about the hip, *Mayo Clin. Proc.*, **59**, 411–14.
Kempf, I., Grosse, A. and Beck, G. (1985) Closed locked intramedullary nailing, *J. Bone Joint Surg.*, (Amer) **67–A**, 709–720.
Dabezies, E. J. S. Ambrosia, R. *et al.* (1984) Fractures of the femoral shaft treated by external fixation using the Wagner Device, *J. Bone Joint Surg.* (Amer) **66–A**, 360–4.
Hardy, A. (1983) Treatment of femoral fractures by cast brace application and early ambulation, prospective review of 106 patients, *J. Bone Joint Surg.*, (Amer) **65–A**, 56–65.

Tibial fractures

Behrens, F. and Searls, K. (1986) External fixation of the tibia : basic concepts and prospective evaluation, *J. Bone Joint Surg.*, (Brit.) **68–B**, 246–54.
Olerud, S. and Kalstrom, G. (1986) The spectrum of intramedullary nailing of the tibia, *Clin. Orthop.*, **212**, 101–112.

FURTHER READING

Shatzker, J. and Tile, M. (1987) *The Rationale of Operative Fracture Care*, Springer-Verlag, Berlin.
Brunner, Ch. F. and Weber, B. G. (1982) *Special Techniques in Internal Fixation*, Springer-Verlag, Berlin.
Weber, B. G. and Cech, O.(1976) *Pseudarthrosis*, Hans Huber, Bern.
Pauwels, F. (1980) *Biomechanics of the Locomotor Apparatus*, Springer-Verlag, Berlin.

CHAPTER FIVE

Complications of specific dislocations

5.1 HAND, WRIST AND ELBOW

5.1.1 DISLOCATIONS OF THE PHALANGES

Finger injuries and dislocations in particular are common on the sporting field. Sports people often reduce these themselves or with the aid of a friend and then strap the finger and carry on playing. However not all dislocations are as friendly and the following are some of the problems.

(i) Irreducible dislocations

This usually occurs when the head of the phalanx buttonholes through the capsule and the capsule then grips around the neck of the phalanx (Fig. 5.1).

TREATMENT _____

Operative treatment is needed and the capsular defect is initially widened (to allow the head to slip back into place) and then repaired. The dislocation when reduced is stable but the finger needs to be protected by splint-age for three weeks. Initially use an aluminium splint and later strap to an adjacent finger and start mobilization.

_____

(ii) Compound dislocations

These are common.

TREATMENT _____

All compound wounds must be carefully cleaned, the wounds debrided and if possible repair carried out. As there is often extensive soft tissue damage the joint may be unstable and may need to be splinted by the insertion of a Kirschner wire after reduction (Fig. 5.2). Dressings and antibiotics and tetanus cover will be needed.

_____

(iii) Fracture dislocations

These are also common and often lead to stiffness, pain and loss of hand function.

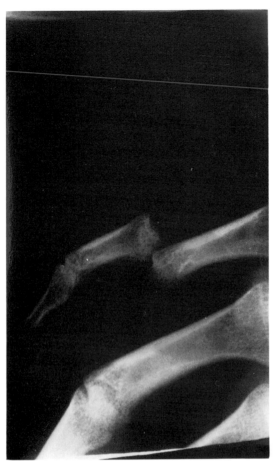

Fig. 5.1 Ventral buttonholing of the head of the proximal phalanx. This dislocation was irreducible.

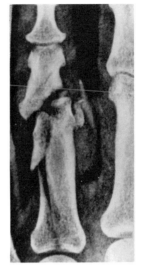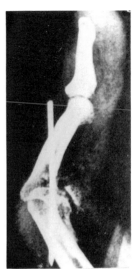

Fig. 5.2 Stabilization of an unstable dislocation with a Kirschner wire.

many of these fracture dislocations although initially reduced will sublux with simple splintage.
b. **Protection of the reduction by insertion of a Kirschner wire across the joint should always be considered.**
c. **Large pieces of articular surfaces if displaced will require reduction and fixation with wires (Fig. 5.3).**

TREATMENT

Reduction and maintenance of the joint and the fracture in good position are the principles of treatment.

KEY POINTS

a. **Often the fracture fragments will be reduced when the dislocation is reduced, but stability is always doubtful and**

(iv) Tendon injuries

These are common in association with dislocations, especially to the extensor mechanism.

TREATMENT

1. **Avulsions of the central slip of the extensor mechanism from the base of the middle phalanx should be repaired or a Bouton-**

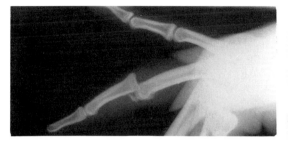

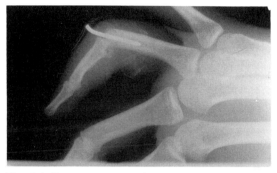

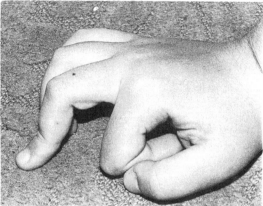

Fig. 5.4 Central slip injury of the extensor tendon leads to a Boutonniere deformity.

Fig. 5.3 Reconstruction of the joint in a fracture dislocation with the aid of Kirschner wires.

niere deformity will result (Fig. 5.4).

2. A Mallet finger deformity (Fig. 5.5) occurs with avulsion of the extensor insertion of the distal phalanx and this requires repair or splintage of the distal phalanx in full extension.

3. Avulsion of the flexor digitorum longus insertion may be missed initially but needs repair.

5.1.2 METACARPOPHALANGEAL DISLOCATIONS

These dislocations are rare and the major problems associated with them are:

(i) Lateral collateral ligament injury

Damage to this ligament may also be associated with an avulsion fracture of either the base of the proximal phalanx (Fig. 5.6) or the head of the metacarpal.

Gamekeeper's thumb Gamekeeper's thumb is an example of this type of lesion, with or without the avulsion fracture. The injury used to occur when the poacher or gamekeeper broke a rabbit or hare's neck forcefully using the thumb web. A chronic instability of the first metacarpophalangeal joint resulted (Fig. 5.7).

TREATMENT

If an avulsion fracture shows displacement of 2–3 mm or rotation of the fragment, open reduction and fixation of the fragment is indicated. Fixation is best carried out by a suture or in the case of a larger fragment, by a small K-wire.

(ii) Irreducible dislocations

Dorsal dislocations can be irreducible due to:

1. Buttonholing of the metacarpal head through the capsule.

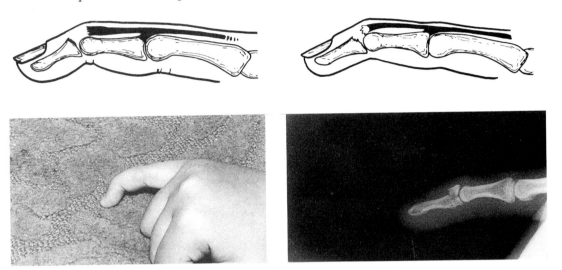

Fig. 5.5 Mallet finger deformity due to the avulsion of the extensor tendon or the piece of bone into which it inserts.

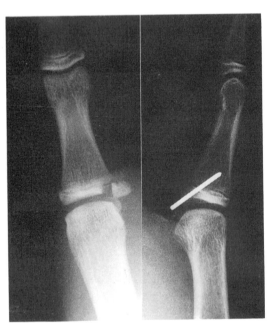

Fig. 5.6 Lateral collateral ligament damage due to avulsion of a bone fragment by abnormal pull on the ligament. Reduction and fixation by Kirschner wire is shown.

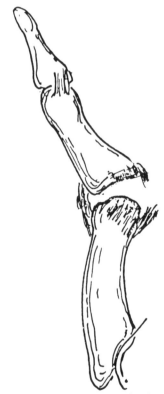

Fig. 5.7 Gamekeeper's or poacher's thumb. A long standing ulnar collateral ligament lesion of the thumb metacarpo-phalangeal joint.

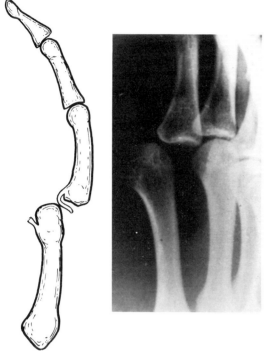

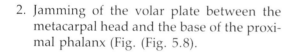

Fig. 5.8 An irreducible dislocation of the metacarpophalangeal joint. Note the volar plate in the joint.

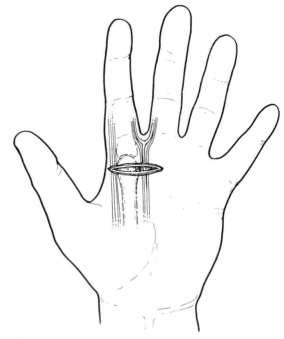

Fig. 5.9 The metacarpal head becomes subcutaneous and pushes the neurovascular bundles anteriorly. Great care needs to be taken during open reduction.

2. Jamming of the volar plate between the metacarpal head and the base of the proximal phalanx (Fig. (Fig. 5.8).

TREATMENT

The volar plate must be removed from the joint and sutured back in place using a volar approach.

┌─ **KEY POINTS** ──────────

Beware of damage to the neurovascular bundles which in these dislocations are just beneath the skin and are stretched tightly across the metacarpal head (Fig. 5.9).

5.1.3 CARPOMETACARPAL DISLOCATIONS OF THE THUMB

This lesion as a pure dislocation is rare (Fig. 5.10). As a fracture dislocation it becomes a Bennett's fracture (Fig. 5.11) and is discussed above.

TREATMENT

This dislocation is easily reduced but is unstable and will require pin fixation for four weeks.

Chronic subluxation of this joint is often seen and in the older patient is often associated with a degenerative arthritis of the carpometacarpal joint of the thumb (Fig. 5.12).

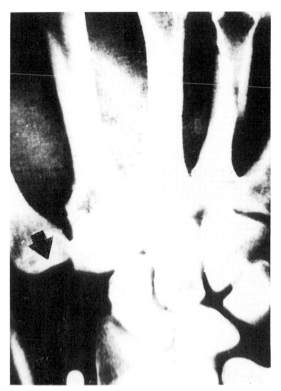

Fig. 5.10 Carpometacarpal dislocation of the thumb, a rare injury.

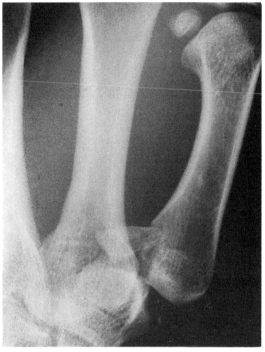

Fig. 5.11 Bennett's fracture dislocation of the carpometacarpal joint of the thumb.

TREATMENT _____

In the younger patient a tenodesis can be successful in stabilizing the joint but in the older patient the accent is on treating the accompanying arthritis with an arthroplasty or an arthrodesis.

_____

5.1.4 DISLOCATIONS OF THE WRIST JOINT

True dislocations of the wrist joint are rare but dislocations of or around the lunate with or without a fracture dislocation of the scaphoid are more common.

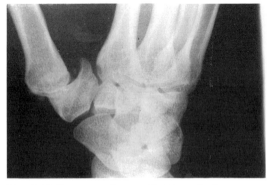

Fig. 5.12 Degenerative arthritis of the carpometacarpal joint of the thumb.

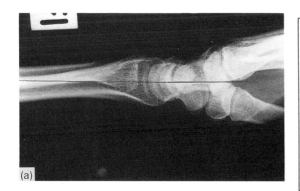

(a)

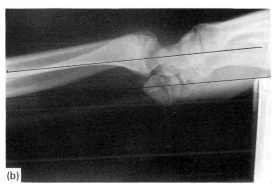

(b)

Fig. 5.13 (a) lateral view of a normal wrist; (b) there is a dislocation of the lunate ventrally. The carpus is in its normal alignment.

(i) Dislocations of the lunate

The lunate is dislocated ventrally and the carpus is in its normal position. The common problems associated with this lesion are:

1. Missing the dislocation

This is usually because the lateral radiograph of the wrist is not inspected carefully. Fig. 5.13(a) and (b) shows (a) normal wrist and (b) dislocated lunate. Note the double line of carpal bones when there is a dislocation.

TREATMENT

The dislocation is usually easy to reduce if seen early. Neglected cases require open reduction.

> ### KEY POINTS
> a. **Use a ventral approach and open up the carpal tunnel as this will prevent an acute carpal tunnel syndome developing postoperatively.**
> b. **The lunate is easily levered back into position and the capsule repaired to give stability.**

2. Median nerve lesions

Acute median nerve lesions at the wrist may be seen in association with this dislocation especially if reduction is delayed. Decompression of the nerve and carpal tunnel is indicated.

(ii) Perilunate dislocations

The lunate is in place on the distal end of the radius and the rest of the carpus is displaced dorsally (Fig. 5.14). Once again recognition of the lesion is the problem. Again there are two layers of carpal bones as in the lunate dislocation but here the lunate has its normal relationship to the distal end of the radius.

TREATMENT

Reduction of the dislocation is easy if the lesion is recognized in the acute phase. Stability is often poor and Kirschner wires should be used to prevent subluxation.

(iii) Perilunate trans-scaphoid dislocations

This injury is similar to the perilunate dislocation except that remaining in normal position are the lunate and the proximal half of the fractured scaphoid bone (Fig. 5.15).

The problems here are:

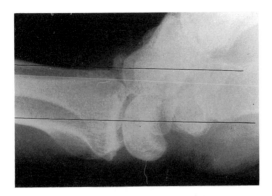

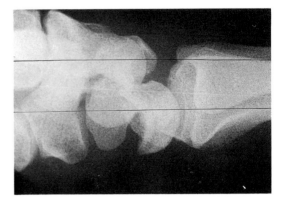

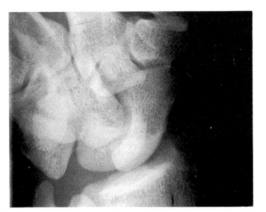

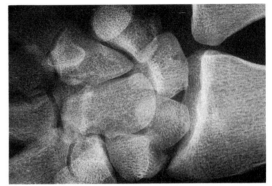

Fig. 5.14 Perilunate dislocation of the carpus. The lunate is in its normal position on the radius, the carpus is dislocated dorsally.

Fig. 5.15 Perilunate transscaphoid dislocation. Here the lunate and half of the scaphoid are in their normal positions.

(a) Recognizing the lesion: Comparative pictures of the various lunate lesions are shown in Fig. 5.16.

(b) Reduction is easy if carried out early but there is such instablity that the fracture of the scaphoid will rarely unite if treated conservatively.

TREATMENT

The fracture of the scaphoid should be treated by internal fixation using a Herbert screw (Fig. 5.17).

KEY POINTS

a. **Use a ventral incision through the posterior aspect of the flexor carpi radialis tendon sheath (Fig. 2.41 and Fig. 2.42).**

b. **Align the scaphoid and apply the special jig which holds the fracture. The screw allows you to drill the hole accurately and tap for the screw of correct length. The screw has the head set in the bone.**

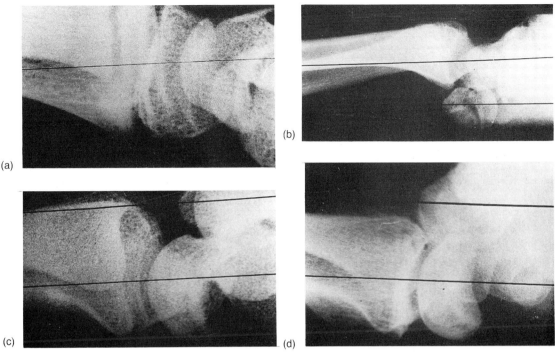

Fig. 5.16 Comparison of the lesions of the carpus: (a) normal carpus, (b) dislocated lunate, (c) perilunate dislocation and (d) perilunate-trans-scaphoid dislocation. The last is difficult to distinguish on the lateral view (which is similar to a perilunate dislocation).

5.1.5 DISLOCATIONS OF THE ELBOW

These are quite common in both children and adults. The complications include:

(i) Missed dislocation
(ii) Irreducible dislocation
(iii) Failure to reduce the head of the radius
(iv) Loss of movement
(v) Calcification and ossification of the capsule and muscles
(vi) Nerve and vascular injury
(vii) Recurrent dislocation

(i) Missed dislocation

It is hard to explain how you can miss a dislocated elbow. It does occur occasionally in the polytraumatized patient and in under-developed countries without medical facilities (Fig. 5.18).

TREATMENT

It is possible to reduce the elbow for up to three weeks after the injury and closed reduction should be tried with prolonged traction under an anaesthetic with relaxation. If this fails then open reduction will be necessary.

KEY POINTS

a. You may need two incisions for this operation.
b. A posterior and lateral incision will allow you to clean out the

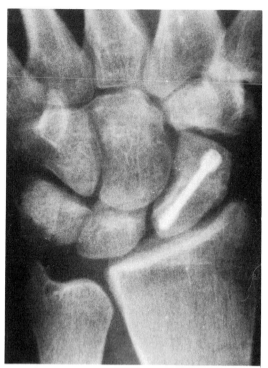

Fig. 5.17 Perilunate trans-scaphoid dislocation treated by reduction of the dislocation and internal fixation using a Herbert screw for the fractured scaphoid.

olecranon fossa and the semilunar notch of the ulna.

c. Traction and gentle levering may now complete the reduction which will be stable at 90 degrees of elbow flexion.

d. If necessary a medial incision over the medial epicondyle and supracondylar ridge can be used to free up the distal end of the humerus anteriorly. However you can generally clear the lower end of the humerus from behind.

e. The medial incision goes down to the bone plane and allows access to the lower end of the humerus anteriorly without endangering the median nerve and the brachial vessels.

(ii) Irreducible dislocation

If you are unable to reduce a dislocated elbow in a child it is because the medial epicondyle is caught in the joint (Fig. 5.19). In an adult it will be due to a fracture with a fragment of bone in the joint. Associated fractures commonly seen in dislocated elbows include osteochondral fragments from the trochlea, and fractures of the coronoid process.

TREATMENT

Open reduction and fixation of the medial epicondyle must be carried out.

┌─ **KEY POINTS** ─

a. **Use a medial incision being careful of the ulnar nerve.**

b. **Identify the ulnar nerve and protect it.**

c. **Dislocate the elbow and remove the epicondyle by following the muscle fibres of the common flexor origin.**

d. **Reduce the dislocation and hold the elbow at 90°**

e. **Pin the epicondyle in place with two Kirschner wires and bend the ends of the wires. You can use a screw in an older child as the epiphysis closes at the age of 15 and there is no deformity if it closes a few years earlier.**

f. **Other loose fragments will need to be removed usually from a lateral approach.**

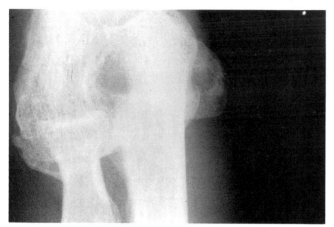

Fig. 5.18 An untreated dislocation of the elbow. Note the calcification in the olecranon fossa.

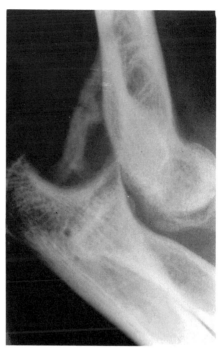

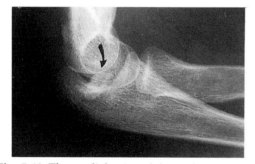

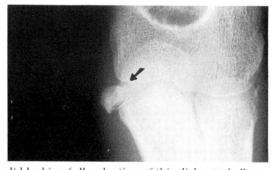

Fig. 5.19 The medial epicondyle can be seen (arrowed) blocking full reduction of this dislocated elbow.

(iii) Failure to reduce the head of the radius

If the head of the radius is still displaced (Fig. 5.20) and the ulna is in place then there must be a fracture of the ulna distally. Occasionally there is only plastic deformation of the ulna (a bend without a break). Fig. 5.21 is a lateral view of a normal elbow for comparison.

TREATMENT

The ulna if fractured must be reduced together with the head of the radius.

Plastic deformation can be corrected by pressure and moulding and of course the head of the radius must be reduced. If the head of the radius is

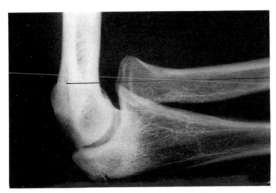

Fig. 5.20 The head of the radius is still dislocated. Compare with Fig. 5.21.

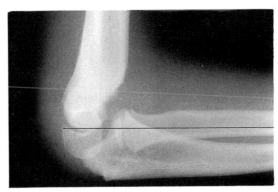

Fig. 5.21 The head of the radius is in its normal position.

unstable then the annular ligament must be reconstructed.

(iv) Loss of movement

This is a common problem in the adult. Most adults who suffer a dislocation of the elbow lose about 20° of extension and about 10° of flexion. Children, particularly the younger ones usually recover fully. It is important to allow time for the capsule to repair and then begin a programme of active movement. Passive stretching of the elbow will increase the scarring and decrease the range of movement. There is no place for passive exercises of the elbow.

(v) Calcification and ossification of the capsule and muscles

Calcification is common in the ligaments and capsule after a dislocation due to the extensive stripping and avulsion. This causes loss of mobility but little else.

Myositis ossificans results from the haematoma that forms in the damaged brachialis muscle and sometimes the triceps becomes ossified. It tends to occur more frequently in those cases associated with severe trauma, repeated attempts at reduction, and passive stretching soon after reduction.

TREATMENT

Once the lesion is established you cannot reverse it. The best you can do is to limit the extent of the lesion by ceasing exercise and allowing the bone to mature. Gross loss of movement occurs. Occasional good results follow delayed excision (1–2 years) of the bone with careful control of bleeding, but generally the results of treatment are disappointing.

(vi) Nerve and vascular injury

These lesions are rare. The commonest nerve injury is a stretching and bruising of the median nerve. The ulna nerve may also be damaged by stretching in fractures. Very rarely the median nerve may actually be trapped in the elbow joint after reduction.

Except for the cases of entrapment, recovery will occur spontaneously over a period of three to twelve weeks and can be monitored by electromyography and return of function. If a nerve fails to show progressive recovery during this time entrapment should be considered and the nerve explored.

Damage to the brachial artery can occur and may be a complete rupture or just intimal damage. The vessel can be trapped in the

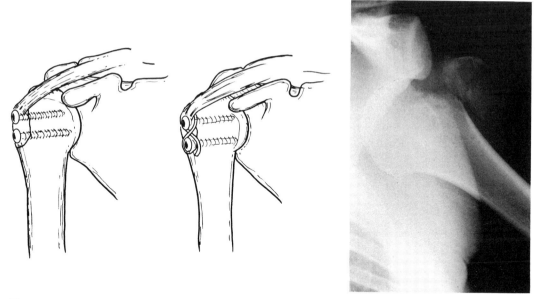

Fig. 5.22 Dislocated shoulder with a displaced fracture of the greater tuberosity. Open reduction and fixation may be necessary.

elbow joint (Fig. 2.80). It is important to recognize the problem early and enlist the help of a vascular surgeon. A vein graft may be necessary.

(vii) Recurrent dislocation

This occurs rarely and is usually associated with a significant fracture of the coronoid process which remains displaced. The anterior capsule must also be deficient.

TREATMENT _____

This is complicated and may include the use of a bone block to deepen the semilunar notch.

5.2 SHOULDER REGION

5.2.1 SHOULDER DISLOCATIONS

These are relatively common injuries especially in body contact sports. Amongst the common complications are:

(i) Associated fracture of the greater tuberosity

This fracture (Fig. 5.22) is almost always reduced into place when the dislocation is reduced and therefore may not need extra treatment. Occasionally the fragment is large and requires to be wired or screwed into place.

TREATMENT _____

The approach for this operation is through the delto—pectoral groove elevating the anterior portion of the deltoid.

(ii) Associated fracture of the glenoid margin

A much rarer fracture/dislocation is the dislocated shoulder with associated fracture of the glenoid margin. This is an unstable situation that demands fixation of the glenoid margin (Fig. 5.23).

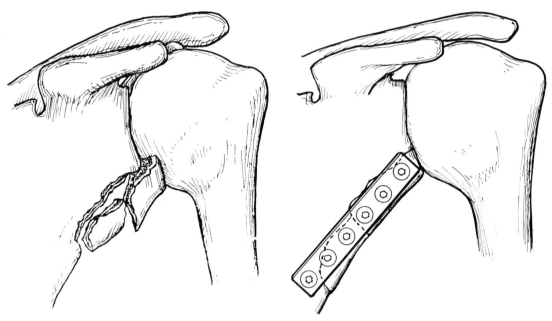

Fig. 5.23 Fracture dislocation with disruption of the inferior glenoid margin often requires internal fixation.

(iii) Further dislocation

Following an initial dislocated shoulder 31% of patients have a further dislocation within two years. The percentage is higher in the younger patient and is almost nil in the over 40 age group. Most of the further dislocations occur during sporting activities. No sporting activities should be allowed for six weeks after a shoulder dislocation.

(iv) Recurrent dislocation (two or more dislocations) is the most common complication of a simple dislocation of the shoulder.

TREATMENT

There are many operative procedures in use for this condition.

The common ones are:

1. The Putti–Platt procedure

KEY POINTS

a. **Delto–pectoral incision, use the cephalic vein as the marker.**
b. **Locate and divide the conjoint tendon 1 cm from its insertion.**
c. **Sweep veins from subscapularis and put in a marker stitch 3 cm from insertion.**
d. **Divide subscapularis and capsule.**
e. **Double breast the capsule and subscapularis. This effectively limits external rotation (Fig. 5.24). This restriction of external rotation persists.**

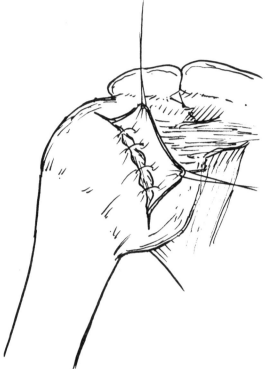

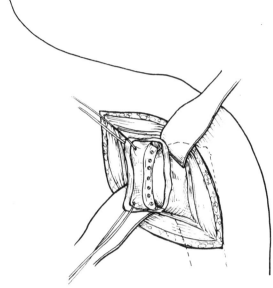

Fig. 5.25 The Bankart operation requires the labrum and capsule to be repaired and reattaching them to the glenoid.

Fig. 5.24 The Putti–Platt procedure requires double breasting of the capsule and subscapularis.

2. The Bankart procedure

┌─ **KEY POINTS** ──────────

a. **Delto–pectoral incision, use the cephalic vein as the marker.**
b. **Locate and divide conjoint tendon 1 cm from insertion.**
c. **Sweep veins from subscapularis and put in a marker stitch 3 cm from insertion.**
d. **Divide subscapularis and the capsule.**
e. **Use an angled retractor to hold back the labrum and capsule which has been stripped (the 'Bankart lesion').**

f. **Use a right angle (dental) drill to make holes in the glenoid margin and suture the labrum back in place (Fig. 5.25).**

3. Boychev's procedure (modified)

┌─ **KEY POINTS** ──────────

a. **Delto–pectoral incision, use the cephalic vein as the marker.**
b. **Locate the conjoint tendon and define the borders down to the penetration of the nerve supply on the medial side.**
c. **Drill and osteotomize the coracoid process half a centimetre from the tip and free the conjoint tendon and muscle down to the nerve supply.**

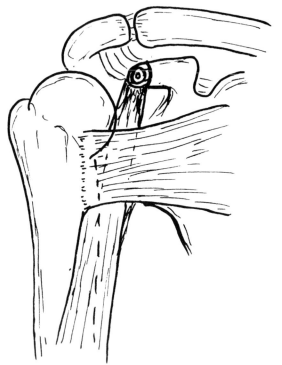

Fig. 5.26 Boychev's operation involves rerouting the conjoint tendon beneath the subscapularis and screwing it back in place.

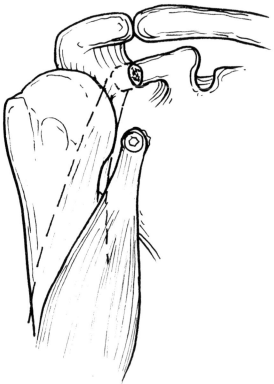

Fig. 5.27 Bristow's operation involves screwing the tip of the coracoid process to the front of the shoulder joint.

4. Bristow's operation

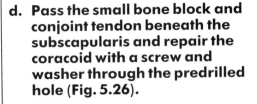

> **d. Pass the small bone block and conjoint tendon beneath the subscapularis and repair the coracoid with a screw and washer through the predrilled hole (Fig. 5.26).**

KEY POINTS

a. **Delto–pectoral incision, use the cephalic vein as the marker.**
b. **Locate the conjoint tendon and drill a hole with a 3.2 mm bit into the coracoid process and then osteotomize the process 1.5 cm from the tip.**
c. **Split the subscapularis and locate the new home for the tip of the coracoid process, slightly below the midpoint of the glenoid labrum, drill the receiving hole and screw home the coracoid process (Fig. 5.27).**

This is the procedure I now use. It is easier that the Putti Platt, which I have also used extensively and does not give an external rotation limitation.

For recurrences, which I see occasionally following operation by someone else, I use Bristow's operation.

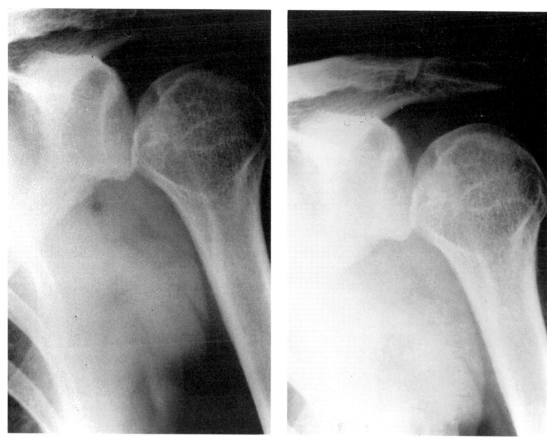

Fig. 5.28 The whole of the glenoid rim is not normally visible. If it is then suspect a posterior dislocation.

(v) Posterior dislocations of the shoulder

This rare injury is often missed by the clinician and occasionally by the radiologist. Medical defence organizations are always reporting actions based on the failure to recognize and treat this injury.

How to idenify the lesion

1. Suspect a posterior dislocation when the whole of the glenoid is visible, normally the humerus blocks the posterior margin giving a half moon effect (Fig. 5.28);
2. Moloney's lines (Fig. 5.29) drawn on the lateral transthoracic radiographs will also confirm the diagnosis;
3. Confirm the posterior dislocation by taking an axillary view of the shoulder (Fig. 5.30);
4. A true axillary lateral radiograph will show the dislocation and the position of the head of the humerus.

Complications are

(a) failure to recognize the lesion
(b) recurrent dislocation

Unrecognized lesions that are unreduced will require open reduction and repair of the posterior structures. Recurrent dislocations can be treated by double breasting the infra-

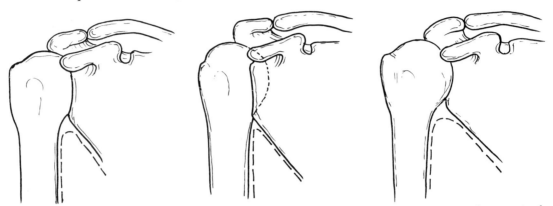

Fig. 5.29 Moloney's lines can be drawn on transthoracic axillary views. Note the smooth curve in the normal shoulder, the sharp acute angle in the posterior dislocation and the broad flat curve in the anterior dislocation.

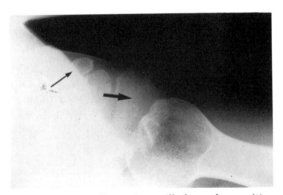

Fig. 5.30 An axillary view will show the position of the head in relation to the glenoid. The broad arrow shows the glenoid and the small arrow the clavicle anteriorly.

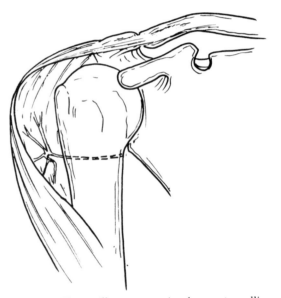

Fig. 5.31 The axillary nerve is shown travelling around the humerus on and in the inferior surface of the deltoid.

spinatus (the so called reverse Putti-Platt operation).

(vi) Nerve injuries

1. The axillary nerve

This is the nerve most commonly injured in association with a dislocated shoulder (Fig. 5.31).

The axillary nerve supplies motor power to the deltoid muscle and a small patch of sensation over the skin at the insertion of the deltoid. (Fig. 5.32).

Sensation returns before motor power and the return of sensation is an excellent prognostic sign.

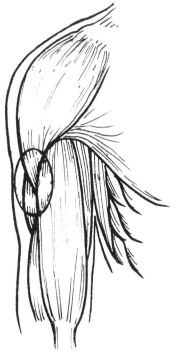

Fig. 5.32 The small area of sensory loss at the insertion of the deltoid in axilllary nerve damage.

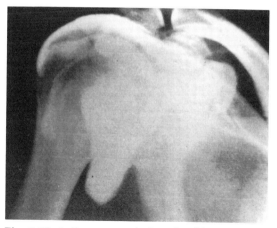

Fig. 5.33 Arthrogram of the shoulder showing leakage of the dye into the subacromial bursa through a tear in the rotator cuff.

TREATMENT

Treatment will not help if the nerve has been avulsed. If there is neuropraxia then there may still be sensation present in the area supplied by the nerve. Recovery of sensation means motor recovery will follow in about three weeks. Over 95% of all cases recover within six months.

Permanent and total paralysis of the deltoid leaves considerable disability. Abduction of the shoulder is only possible to 30–40° in. Arthrodesis of the shoulder joint will allow better function of the upper limb (Fig. 2.118).

2. Other nerve injuries

These are much less common. The musculo–cutaneous nerve and the median nerve can be damaged. Full recovery can be expected. Traction injuries to the brachial plexus also (rarely) occur, their prognosis is not good.

(vii) Rotator cuff lesions

The rotator cuff is often damaged in dislocations and this can be demonstrated clinically and by arthrogram (Fig. 5.33). Repair is not necessary.

(viii) Missed dislocation

There are occasions especially in elderly people when a dislocation of the shoulder is missed for days or weeks. Reduction then is sometimes possible but there are two problems that can occur:

1. If you use too much force (especially in a rotary plane), you can get a spiral fracture of upper third of the shaft or a fracture of the neck of the humerus as well as an unreduced dislocation (Fig. 5.34).
2. You can damage the axillary vessels.

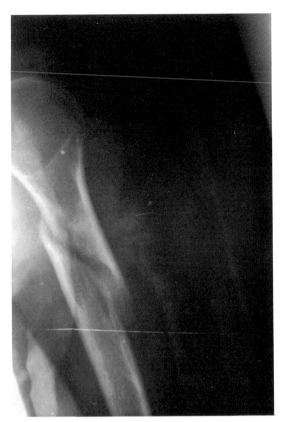

Fig. 5.34 Spiral fracture of the upper third of the humerus after attempts to reduce a dislocated shoulder.

TREATMENT

Both the above are disastrous complications and can be avoided with care. It is always worthwhile trying a gentle closed reduction under anaesthesia with firm and prolonged traction. No violence should be used. If this is not successful then open reduction will be necessary.

The basic rule with dislocations of the shoulder should be that if the dislocation cannot be reduced with gentle manoeuvres under analgesia then reduction under anaesthesia should be done. If the shoulder cannot be reduced under anaesthesia then open reduction is necessary.

(ix) Vascular problems

These can occur at the time of dislocation or during reduction especially if it is violent. The patient is usually elderly. If there is arterial damage the axilla rapidly becomes distended and painful, the hand pale, cyanotic and cold. There is often numbness in the arm and hand. The axillary artery and/or vein may be completely ruptured or one of its branches avulsed. The patient may be shocked. Thrombosis of the artery can also occur.

TREATMENT

The vessels must be restored by direct repair or replacement, or bypass.

5.2.2 ACROMIOCLAVICULAR DISLOCATIONS

These dislocations occur commonly and are usually the result of a fall on the point of the shoulder. Complications are rare and consist mainly of:

(i) Gross deformity in complete dislocations (Fig. 5.35).
(ii) Pain due to impingement at the joint

(i) Gross deformity

Complete dislocation means there is disruption of the trapezoid and conoid ligaments (Fig. 5.35) which run from the coracoid to the inferior surface of the clavicle and are basically responsible for the stability of the outer end of the clavicle. The distal end of the clavicle rides out of the acromio–clavicular articulation and forms an ugly prominence.

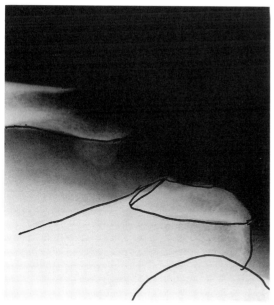

Fig. 5.35 Gross displacement and deformity of the acromio-clavicular joint.

TREATMENT

Complete dislocations of the clavicle should be stabilized in the reduced position to allow healing of the coraco—clavicular ligaments.

shown in Fig. 5.36. The one I favour is the simplest, the use of heavy wires (heavy Kirschner wires or small Steinman's pins) inserted through the acromion and across the joint. The coraco—clavicular screw is probably the most frequently used method.

c. The pin must be bent over into a U shape and the end buried in the bone. This prevents migration into and through the neck (**Fig. 5.37**) or protrusion through the skin. A tension band wire can be added as support.

d. Surgical repair of the torn ligaments or reinforcement of the ligaments with the coraco—acromial ligament is advocated by some, however if the reduction and pinning is carried out within a few days of the injury it is not necessary.

e. In late cases it is necessary to excise the outer end of the clavicle and to hold down the clavicle with a ligamentous repair. I use the dorsal periosteum and suture it firmly to remnants of the ligaments in the bed of the excised clavicular segment.

KEY POINTS

a. There are a number of ways of stabilizing the joint operatively whilst the ligaments heal. A sling will support an incomplete lesion but not a total dislocation. Strapping is uncomfortable and useless.

b. Operations commonly used are

Complications after internal fixation of this injury include:

1. Wound infection
2. Breakage of wires (Fig. 5.38)
3. Migration of wires
4. Pulling out of the 'Bosworth screw'
5. Fracture of the coracoid process of the scapula

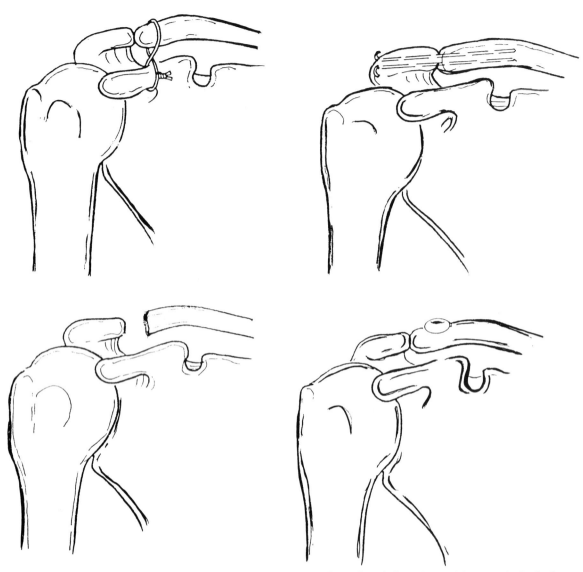

Fig. 5.36 The various common operations for acromioclavicular dislocations: (a) acromioclavicular loop; (b) heavy wires across the joint; (c) excision of the outer end of the clavicle; (d) Bosworth claviculo–coracoid screw.

(ii) Pain due to impingement

Pain after damage to the acromioclavicular joint occurs after both subluxation and frank dislocation. The pain is well localized and occurs at nearly full abduction or elevation. It is relieved temporarily by injecting local anaesthetic into the joint.

TREATMENT

Excision of the outer end of the clavicle gives dramatic results but the clavicle must be held down in cases of complete dislocation.

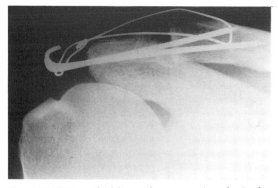

Fig. 5.37 Wires holding the acromio–clavicular joint must be heavy and have the ends bent over to stop penetration.

and is useful for repair and filling the defect.

c. **Excise a generous 2 cm of the clavicle using a sharp osteotome. Do not point the osteotome anteriorly or inferiorly as the subclavian vessels and the lung are not far away should the instrument slip.**
d. **Fully abduct the arm and make sure there is plenty of room between the shortened clavicle and the acromion. Use the periosteum to hold down the clavicle as described above or to fill the gap.**

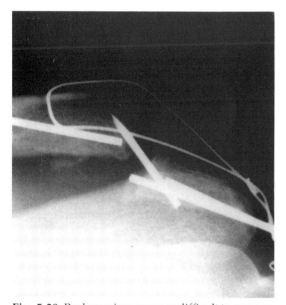

Fig. 5.38 Broken wires are very difficult to remove.

5.2.3 STERNOCLAVICULAR DISLOCATIONS

These injuries are fortunately rare as they are frequently troublesome. The complications include:

(i) Obstruction of the trachea
(ii) Difficulties in reduction
(iii) Difficulties in maintaining the reduction
(iv) Long term cosmetic deformity and pain

(i) Obstruction of the trachea

In a posterior dislocation (Fig. 5.39) the medial end of the clavicle can obstruct the trachea and or press on the great vessels in the mediastinum. Reduction can be a matter of extreme urgency and lives have been lost on the football field with this injury.

KEY POINTS

a. **Use a sabre cut incision.**
b. **Preserve the dorsal periosteum, as it is thickened**

TREATMENT

Almost all these dislocations will reduce if the patients shoulders are pulled back and gentle pressure ap-

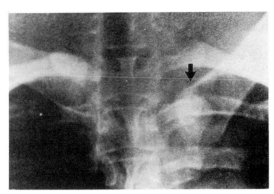

Fig. 5.39 Posterior sternoclavicular dislocation.

plied with a knee in between the scapulae. The shoulders will need to be kept back in a figure of eight bandage or a harness for three to four weeks (Fig. 3.5).

(ii) Difficulties in reduction

This can occur in both posterior and anterior dislocations especially if there has been some delay since the original injury. If closed reduction as described above is unsuccessful, then use a towel clip with sharp points to grip the clavicle and pull it forward whilst the shoulders are pulled back.

(iii) Difficulties in maintaining the reduction

This occurs mainly in the anterior dislocation of the sterno-clavicular joint. Some degree of subluxation should be accepted rather than use wires across this joint. **Do not use wires. Do not use wires.** There have been charges of **murder** against two surgeons who used wires that migrated to the heart and killed the patients.

(iv) Cosmetic deformity and pain

Cosmetic deformity and some discomfort are common sequelae of anterior dislocations but the functional impairment is slight. Rarely excision of the medial end of the clavicle is indicated to relieve pain localized to this joint (Fig. 5.40). This localization should be confirmed by the relief of pain after injection of local anaesthetic into the joint. If excision is carried out then it must be confined to those cases which have an intact costoclavicular ligament, and excision must be medial to this ligament.

5.3 HIP

Dislocations of the hip are major injuries and are often associated with complications.

The major complications include:

   (i) Difficulty with closed reduction
  (ii) Associated fractures
 (iii) Central dislocation
 (iv) Nerve injury
  (v) Avascular necrosis of the head of the femur
 (vi) Myositis ossificans
(vii) Unsuspected knee ligament damage
(viii) Traumatic arthritis

(i) Difficulty with closed reduction

Most dislocations of the hip are reduced by closed methods such as the Allis method shown in Fig. 5.41, or the foot in groin method shown in Fig. 5.42.

If you have the patient under a relaxant anaesthetic then muscle spasm is not a problem, so that if there is difficulty in reducing a dislocated hip one of the following may be the cause:

(a) Button holing of the dislocated head through a small tear in the capsule which stretches over the head and then grips tightly around the neck of the femur.
(b) A piece of the posterior acetabular wall is being pulled into the joint before the head of the femur (Fig. 5.43).
(c) A piece of the head of the femur has been

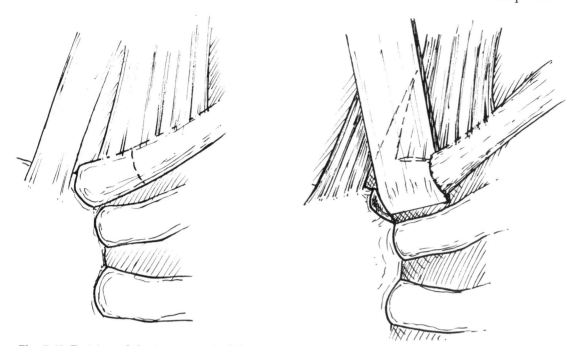

Fig. 5.40 Excision of the innner end of the clavicle. Protect the posterior structures.

broken away and is jamming the joint (Fig. 5.44).

TREATMENT

Open reduction of the dislocation is essential to overcome any block to reduction.

KEY POINTS

a. **Most dislocations (and therefore most irreducible dislocations) are posterior, hence you should use a posterior approach such as the Southern approach of Austin Moore (Fig. 5.45).**

b. **If the irreducible dislocation is anterior the the incision should be a Smith-Petersen approach (Fig. 5.46).**

c. **Care needs to be taken when using the Southern approach to identify the sciatic nerve and to protect it.**

d. **The capsule has to be opened widely and the block to reduction removed.**

e. **The fractures associated with the dislocation need to be dealt with (see below).**

(ii) Associated fractures

1. Posterior acetabular wall

Fractures of the posterior wall of the acetabulum are frequently associated with posterior dislocations of the hip (Fig. 5.47).

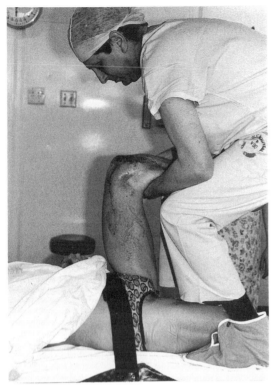

Fig. 5.41 The Allis method of reduction of a dislocated hip.

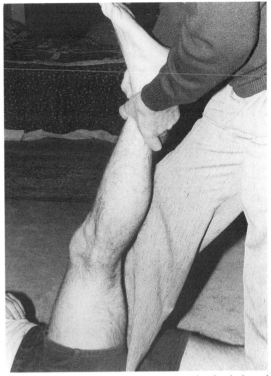

Fig. 5.42 The foot in the groin method of closed reduction of a dislocated hip.

Their importance is that:

(a) If the fragment is large the hip will be unstable and will tend to dislocate or subluxate.
(b) The fragment may reduce into the joint cavity before the head and be a block to reduction (see above).
(c) As this is an intra-articular fracture the joint is more likely to be damaged and develop into a traumatic arthritis.

TREATMENT

Small fragments (those of a few millimetres) can be ignored. Larger fragments need to be openly reduced

and held in place with screws (Fig. 5.48).

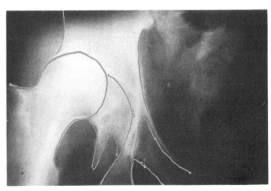

Fig. 5.43 A large piece of acetabulum is in the joint.

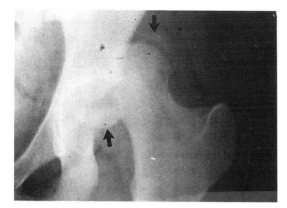

Fig. 5.44 A piece of the head of the femur is in the joint.

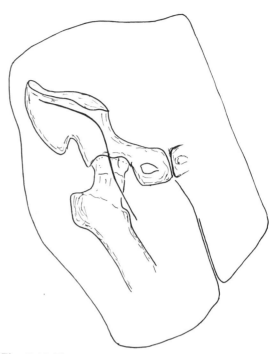

Fig. 5.46 The anterior 'Smith-Petersen' approach.

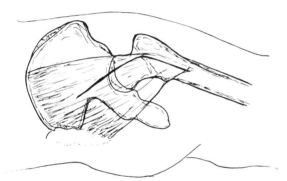

Fig. 5.45 The 'Southern' approach to the hip joint.

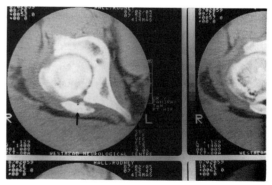

Fig. 5.47 Large fragment has been detatched from the posterior acetabular wall as seen on this CT scan.

KEY POINTS

a. **Use a posterior approach and protect the sciatic nerve.**
b. **Reduce the fragment and hold with a Kirschner wire whilst the screw hole is drilled and tapped.**
c. **Take care with the direction of the screw to be sure that you do not go into the hip joint or the head of the femur.**

---

2. Femoral head

Fractures of the head of the femur associated with dislocations of the head of the femur present problems for the following reasons:

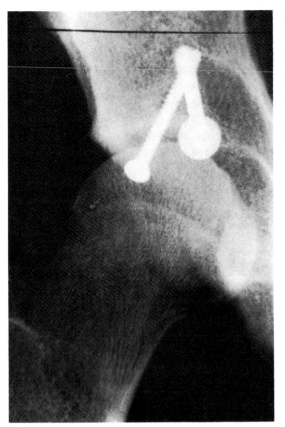

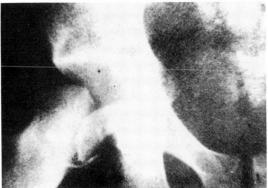

Fig. 5.49 Large segment of the inferior part of the head of the femur has broken away and is free in the hip joint and will block reduction.

Fig. 5.48 Open reduction and screw fixation of the posterior acetabular fragment restores joint stability and congruity.

(a) The fracture is always a significant one and can involve a large piece of articular surface (Fig. 5.49).

(b) There is a very high incidence of the fragment jamming in the joint during reduction.

(c) Almost all these joints go on to a traumatic arthritis.

TREATMENT

Open reduction and either fixation of the fragment with a screw such as a Herbert screw (which is automatically countersunk below the articular surface), or excision of the fragment.

┌─── **KEY POINTS** ───────────┐

a. This is a difficult procedure and needs wide exposure.

b. Wherever possible preserve any attachments of soft tissue or capsule to the fragment (to preserve the blood supply).

└──────────────────────────────┘

(iii) Central dislocation

This lesion in its worst form has the head of the femur poking through the floor of the acetabulum (Fig. 5.50) and lying in the pelvic cavity with both the anterior and posterior pelvic columns broken (Fig. 5.51). The shaft of the femur is hard up against the labrum acetabulare.

The lesser forms of the fracture dislocation have some disruption of the pelvic floor with some medial shift of the head of the femur and in these cases only one of the columns of the pelvis is broken (Fig. 5.52).

Problems encountered with central dislocation of the hip include the following:

1. Associated pelvic injuries, such as injuries to the bladder, or pelvic vessels.

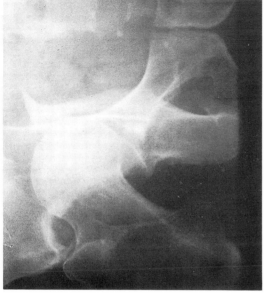

Fig. 5.50 Central dislocation of the hip.

TREATMENT

Laparotomy and repair of damage to the bladder and other pelvic organs is essential. If the patient's condition after this repair is satisfactory, reduction and fixation of the pelvic fracture may be carried out through the laparotomy incision. (It is of course not advisable if bowel surgery has been necessary.)

2. Difficulties in reduction and maintenance of the floor of the acetabulum.

TREATMENT

There are two ways to treat a central dislocation:

1. **By lateral traction in the line of the neck of the femur by a Green screw or similar device (Fig. 5.53). If you adopt this method the reduction must be complete and the alignment must be maintained by traction for at least six weeks to allow union of the acetabular floor. If you fail to obtain reduction of the pelvic floor then carry out open reduction and fixation of the pelvic fracture.**

2. **By open reduction and fixation to restore the floor of the acetabulum. This procedure is not easy and one should be prepared to internally fix both the anterior and posterior columns of the pelvis depending on the type of fracture (Fig. 5.54).**

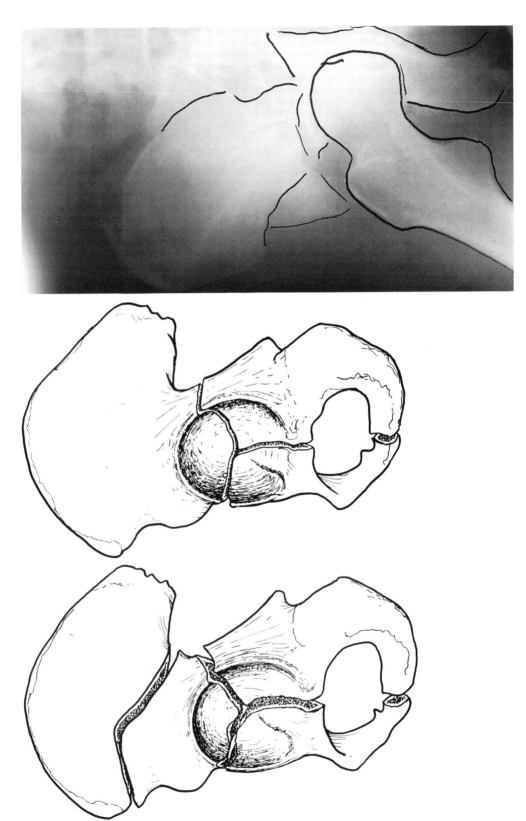

Fig. 5.51 The pelvic fracture in a central dislocation.

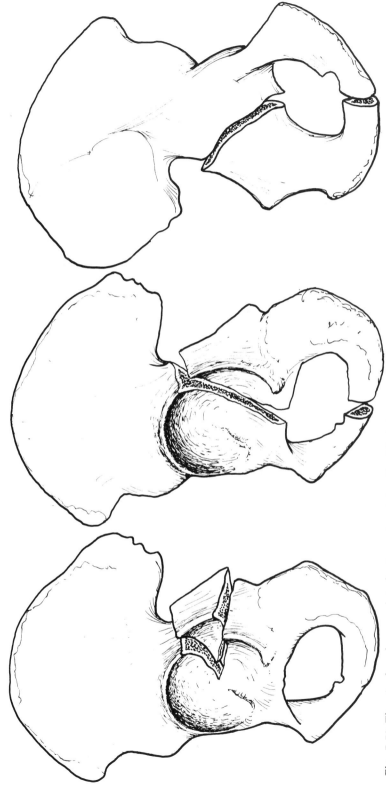

Fig. 5.52 The single column pelvic fractures involving the hip joint.

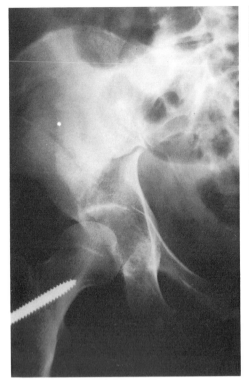

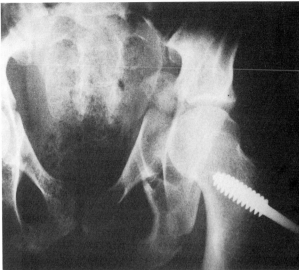

Fig. 5.53 Lateral traction through a Green screw.

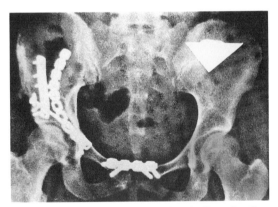

Fig. 5.54 Pelvic reconstruction including the floor of the acetabulum.

KEY POINTS

a. It is essential that there is good visualization of the fracture on radiographs. CT scans can help but all the information is available on anteroposteror, obturator and iliac views.

b. Numerous approaches have been advocated but there is no incision which suits all fractures of the pelvis. You may need to approach the anterior and posterior columns separately.

c. You will need to have special plates, flexible drive drills and taps and flexible drive screwdrivers (**Fig. 5.55**).

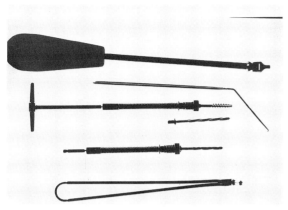

Fig. 5.55 Flexible screwdriver and drills enable you to work at unusual angles and in confined spaces.

3. Pin tract infection and osteomyelitis can occur through the Green screw and into the greater trochanter region. Osteomyelitis will need to be treated by drainage and removal of sequestra under suitable antibiotic cover.

(iv) Nerve injury

The sciatic nerve can be damaged in a posterior dislocation. The nerve can also be damaged during operative procedures and due care needs to be taken to identify and protect the nerve (see above) especially when the posterior or 'Southern' approach is used.

The lateral popliteal division tends to be more severely affected giving a foot drop. The nerve damage can be due to:

1. Stretching during the actual dislocation (the lesion should be detected before reduction).
2. Damage by a fragment of the posterior rim of the acetabulum. A sharp fragment can cut the nerve.
3. Damage during closed or open reduction (i.e. working before reduction but not after reduction).
4. Delayed onset due to the nerve being caught in callus.

In most cases the nerve is contused and some recovery can be anticipated within three months. This is especially the case in closed reduction in 1. and 3. above.

TREATMENT

Nerve lesions that do not improve clinically or on electomyography after three months (about 30% of nerve injuries) warrant exploration and freeing of the nerve and in the case of a cut nerve, microsurgical repair. The prognosis is not good but the alternative is to use an orthosis or perform a tendon transfer (see lateral popliteal nerve damage above).

Both the femoral and obturator nerve can be damaged by an anterior dislocation of the hip (Fig. 5.56). These lesions tend to be bruising and stretching and almost invariably recover within three months. Damage may also occur to the femoral vessels in an anterior dislocation of the hip.

(v) Avascular necrosis of the head of the femur

About 6% of dislocations insult the head of the femur sufficiently to cause avascular necrosis of the head and these hips will become painful and arthritic (Fig. 5.57). The diagnosis does not become obvious for some months on the plain films but a nuclear scan will show loss of uptake of the radionuclide.

TREATMENT

There is little that can be carried out once the head becomes avascular except to keep the patient non-weight bearing for about six months to allow revascularization. The problem then

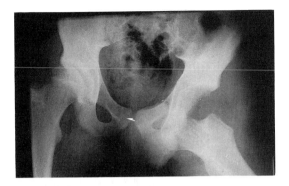

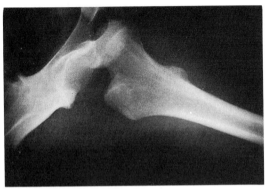

Fig. 5.56 Anterior dislocations of the hip.

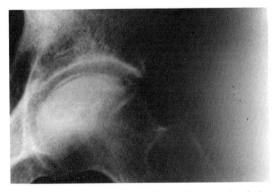

Fig. 5.57 Avascular necrosis of the head of the femur.

becomes one of treatment of a painful arthritic hip which inevitably follows some time later (see below).

(vi) Myositis ossificans

Ossification in the haematoma and of the capsule of the hip joint can occur after dislocations and may be severe enough to limit movement. Excision of mature bone may be indicated.

(vii) Unsuspected knee ligament damage

This is another example of overlooking damage because our attention is drawn to the obvious and major lesion. It stands to reason that if the force that dislocates the hip is transmitted through the knee joint then damage to knee ligaments can occur. In particular always suspect and check for damage to the cruciate ligaments.

(viii) Traumatic arthritis

The incidence of traumatic arthritis after dislocation of the hip depends on three factors:

1. The age of the patient
2. The type of dislocation (i.e. whether associated with a fracture of the acetabulum or femoral head)
3. The timing and ease of reduction

Basically, the simple dislocation in a young person that is easily and atraumatically reduced without delay is least likely to develop arthritis. It is most common with dislocations with fractures of the head of the femur. Arthritis may develop as late as twenty years after a dislocation.

TREATMENT

Traumatic arthritis (Fig. 5.58) presents problems mainly because the patients are often in a younger age

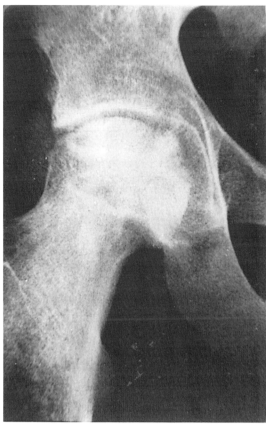

Fig. 5.58 An arthritic hip ten years after a dislocation.

group in which one would he hesitant to advise total hip replacement.

5.4 KNEE JOINT

5.4.1 KNEE JOINT

(Do not confuse with dislocations of the patella (see later).)

Dislocations of the knee joint are horrific injuries.

The complications include:

(i) Major compound wounds
(ii) Major vascular damage
(iii) Severe ligamentous damage
(iv) Damage to the lateral popliteal nerve

(i) Major compound wounds

Compound wounds will need to be treated by the usual protocol of extensive cleaning, debridement, partial closure if at all, splintage and antibiotic and antitetanus cover (see compound wounds in the earlier section).

(ii) Major vessel damage

Major vessel damage is present in about half of the cases of dislocated knee joint. It is more

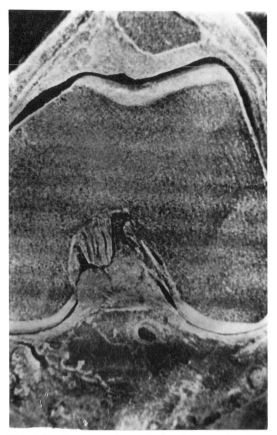

Fig. 5.59 Cross section of the leg at the knee showing the proximity of the vessels.

common when the femur is displaced posteriorly on the tibia. This is hardly surprising when you realize how closely the popliteal vessels are applied to the back of the knee joint (Fig. 5.59).

Damage to the vessels will be obvious from bleeding if there is open wound and from the lack of blood supply distal to the lesion. In closed cases an arteriogram will identify the level of the lesion (Fig. 5.60).

TREATMENT

This is a surgical emergency and the help of a vascular surgeon should be sought without delay. Even with energetic treatment a significant number of these lesions go on to amputation. A vein graft is usually necessary when there is arterial damage.

(iii) Severe ligamentous damage

Ligamentous injuries are common in dislocations of the knee but surprisingly may be incomplete.

TREATMENT

These injuries should be repaired if the vascular status of the leg is satisfactory after reduction. Lesions treated conservatively usually end up with quite a lot of laxity in the knee but reasonable function for quiet use.

(iv) Damage to the lateral popliteal nerve

This is usually caused by traction and very often permanent loss of dorsiflexion of the foot is the result.

TREATMENT

If ligamentous repair is carried out on the lateral side then the nerve should be explored in cases where there is evidence of damage. Often the nerve will look like a piece of soggy spaghetti and there is nothing that can be carried out. Sometimes the nerve is completely avulsed. Wherever possible the nerve should be decompressed. Residual foot drop should be treated with an orthosis or tendon transfers (see lateral popliteal nerve injury above).

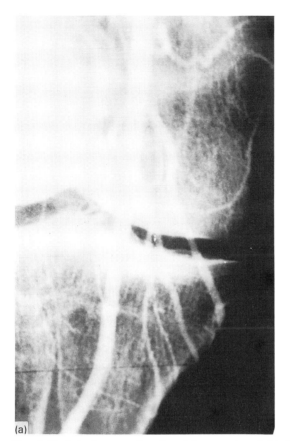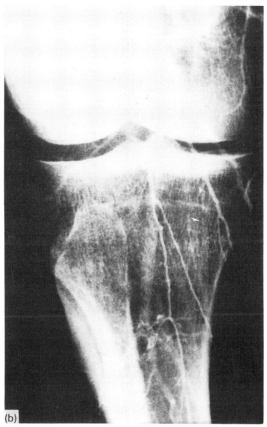

Fig. 5.60 Arteriogram showing (a) normal and (b) damaged and blocked politeal artery.

5.4.2 PATELLA

These dislocations are common. The complications include:

(i) Recurrent dislocation
(ii) Arthritis
(iii) Instability due to anatomical abnormalities

(i) Recurrent dislocation

About 75% of patella dislocations recur and with each further dislocation damage to the medial insertion of the quadriceps and the articular surface increases. Recurrent dislocation of the patella is often associated with abnormalities of the shape of the patella and of the lateral condyle of the femur.

TREATMENT

Proximal realignment of the patella is the most commonly performed of many procedures (Fig. 5.61).

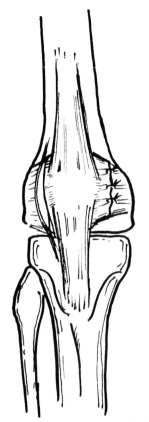

Fig. 5.61 Proximal realignment of the patella, medial plication and lateral release.

(ii) Arthritis

Damage to the articular surface must occur each time the patella dislocates or even subluxes. This alone is a valid reason for operation in recurrent dislocation. The damage may be:

1. To the articular cartilage leading to fibrillation and a frank chondromalacia with retropatellar knee pain with activities such as running and going up and down stairs. (Fig. 5.62).
2. An osteochondral fracture.

TREATMENT

Both these lesions can be assessed arthroscopically. Osteochondral fractures require either removal if small or replacement and fixation if large. At the same time the patella must be realigned, and in the case of severe chondromalacia the insertion of the patella tendon into the tibia may require elevation by a Maquet or an Elmslie-Trillat procedure (Fig. 5.63).

Frank patello–femoral arthritis which is localized to this part of the knee can develop as a result of recurrent dislocation of the patella.

TREATMENT

It is important to be certain that the arthritis is localized to the patello–femoral region, so that arthroscopic examination of the knee is essential. If localized arthritis is confirmed, then at present patellectomy is advised.

KEY POINTS

a. **Perform a full release of the retinaculum and capsule laterally.**
b. **The vastus medialis insertion has to be advanced distally and attached firmly to the medial border of the patella. (In acute cases the insertion is torn away and then heals with a gap.)**
c. **Protect the repair for four weeks.**

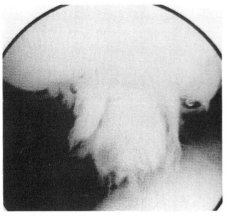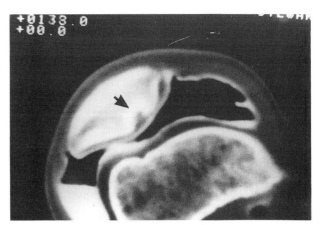

Fig. 5.62 Fibrillation and articular damage to the patella after several dislocations.

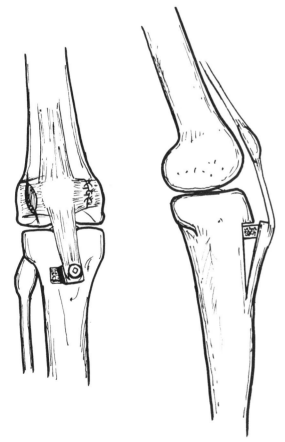

Fig. 5.63 Two methods of realignment of the patella with anterior displacement to relieve the pressure on the patella.

(iii) Instability due to anatomical abnormalities

Abnormalities of the patella and of the lateral femoral condyle can be gross and require treatment. The patella can be small and very high and not sit in the sulcus (patella alta) (Fig. 5.64). On rare occasions the lateral supracondylar ridge is not developed and hence there is nothing to stop the patella sliding laterally.

TREATMENT _____

Severe cases of patella alta where the patella cannot be realigned may warrant patellectomy (see patella fractures for operative details). Elevation of the lateral supracondylar ridge is indicated where this is deficient. A bone block will be needed to support the elevated ridge.

_____

5.4.3 HEAD OF THE FIBULA

This is a rare injury usually caused by a direct blow. The head of the fibula is often but not always dislocated posteriorly.

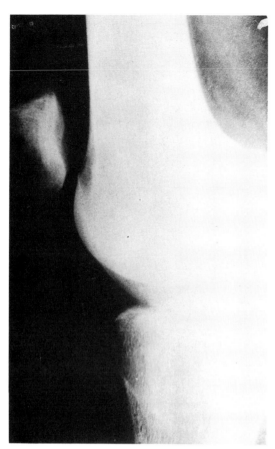

Fig. 5.64 Patella alta, a small high riding patella.

The major problems with this injury are:

1. Instability of the head of the fibula
2. Lateral popliteal nerve injury

TREATMENT

The head of the fibula should be re-located by closed means and if it is unstable held in place with Kirschner wires. If the lateral popliteal nerve shows signs of damage it should be explored and decompressed.

5.5 ANKLE REGION

5.5.1 ANKLE

Most dislocations of the ankle involve fractures and are dealt with in section 4.2.4 on ankle fractures. Rarely there are dislocations of the ankle without fractures as seen in Fig. 5.65.

Complications include:

1. Irreducible dislocation
2. Ligamentous damage

TREATMENT

Irreducible dislocations are usually due to locking of the talus on its side. Open reduction and levering the talus into place is not difficult. Ligamentous damage warrants repair, although some advocate simple plaster immobilizaiton (after reduction) for a period of eight weeks.

5.5.2 TALUS

Dislocations associated with fractures have already been discussed under fractures of the talus (see 4.3.1 (ii)). Talar dislocations may be total as shown in Fig. 5.66 or subtalar (i.e. at the distal talocalcaneal and talonavicular joints).

Complications include:

(i) Irreducible dislocations
(ii) Damage to the joints with pain and stiffness
(iii) Avascular necrosis of the talus

(i) Irreducible dislocations

TREATMENT

Irreducible dislocations are more common in lateral subtalar dislocations and require open reduction and

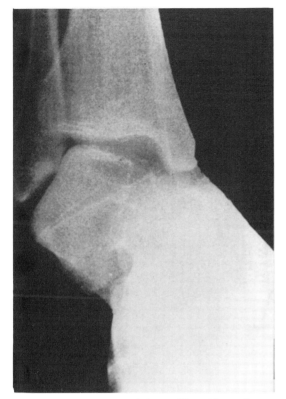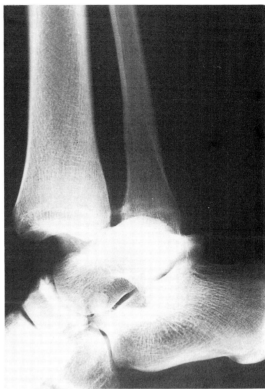

Fig. 5.65 Dislocation of the ankle without fracture, a rare injury.

levering free the locked condyles. The reduction is stable and the patient requires plaster immobilization for four weeks.

Total dislocation of the talus will often be associated with a compound wound that requires debridement and later repair. (Occasionally the talus is found in the patient's sock or at the roadside.) If there is no wound then the skin will be under threat because there is insufficient room for the dislocated talus.

Closed reduction of a total dislocation of the talus is usually unsuccessful and open reduction should be carried out without delay. The talus may be unstable after reduction and

if so a Kirschner wire should be used to provide stability.

(ii) Damage to the joints

Damage to the joints involved in these violent injuries is always great and there will always be stiffness and loss of movement. Loss of inversion and eversion and pain and discomfort on walking on rough ground or running are common symptoms.

(iii) Avascular necrosis

This will not be obvious on plain radiographs for six to eight weeks but a bone scan will

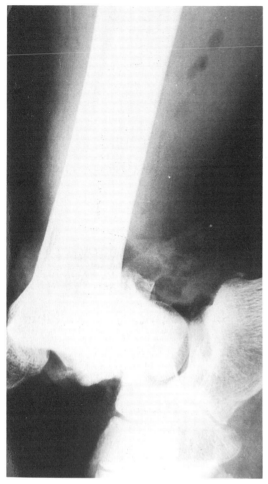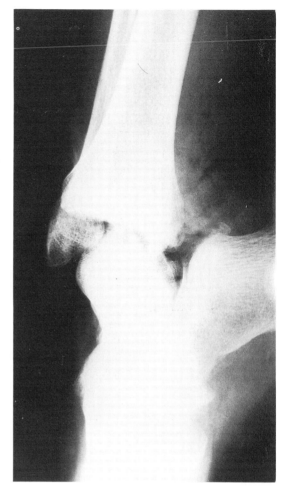

Fig. 5.66 Complete dislocation of the talus.

show the loss of blood supply (see fractures of the talus).

TREATMENT

Avascular necrosis will revascularize in time. A patellar tendon bearing weight relieving orthosis should be used for as long as it takes for the bone to revascularize (this may be as long as two years).

Joints that are painful and are not helped by the usual conservative measures (weight reduction, activity restriction, analgesics and anti-inflammatory drugs) may warrant arthrodesis.

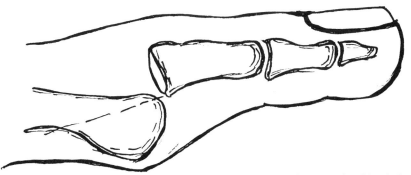

Fig. 5.67 Buttonholing of the metatarsal head is the usual cause of an irreducible dislocation of the metatarso-phalangeal joint.

5.6 FOOT

5.6.1 METATARSO–PHALANGEAL JOINTS

These are similar to the corresponding dislocations in the hand in that they may be simple dislocations or dislocations that are irreducible. The metatarsal head can be trapped by the transverse metatarsal ligament and plantar capsule. The collateral ligaments and the short flexors and intrinsics (Fig. 5.67) tightly grasp the neck of the metatarsal.

TREATMENT _____

Simple dislocations require closed reduction and splinting whereas irreducible dislocations require open reduction.

> **KEY POINTS** ─────
>
> a. **Use a plantar transverse incision.**
> b. **Take care to avoid the neurovascular bundle which can be very superficial.**

> c. **Lever the head back into position after removing the entrapped capsule.**
> d. **If the joint is unstable use a Kirschner wire to stabilize the joint for three weeks.**

5.6.2 INTERPHALANGEAL JOINTS

These dislocations are common but seldom cause problems. Occasionally you come across a neglected dislocation or a joint that remains painful after reduction (Fig. 5.68).

TREATMENT _____

Missed dislocations and painful joints after reduction require arthrodesis of the joint.

> **KEY POINTS** ─────
>
> (a) **Use a dorsal incision and remember that the joints lie a little distal to the creases.**
> (b) **Excise the joint surfaces at an angle that will correct any deformity.**

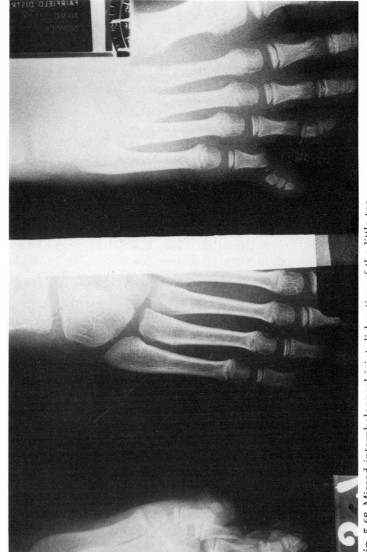

Fig. 5.68 Missed interphalangeal joint dislocation of the little toe.

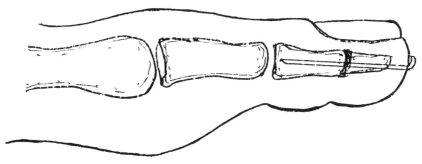

Fig. 5.69 Arthrodesis of a small joint. Excision of the joint surfaces and then fixation with a pin or screw.

(c) Use a Kirschner wire to stabilize the joint. Bend the end of the wire at right angles or greater. The end can be buried or left exposed so that it can be removed without anaesthesia in six weeks when the joint has arthrodesed (Fig.5.69).

FURTHER READING

Rockwood, C.A. and Green, D. P. (1984) *Fractures in Adults*, J. B. Lippincott, Philadelphia.

Wright, P.E., Edmondson, A. S. and Crenshaw, A. H. (1980) *Campbells Operative Orthopaedics*, 6th edn, C. V. Mosby, St. Louis.

Shoulder dislocations

Bankart, A. S. B. (1939) The pathology and treatment of recurrent dislocation of the shoulder joint, *Br. J. Surg.* **26**, 23–9.

Helfet, A. J. (1958) Coracoid transplantation for recurring dislocation of the shoulder. *J. Bone Joint Surg.*, (Br), **40–B**, 198–202.

Boytchev, B. (1951) Operative treatment of recurrent dislocation of the shoulder. *Minerva Orthopedica*, **2**, 377–9.

Hip dislocations

Epstein, H. C. (1980) *Traumatic dislocation of the hip*. Williams and Wilkins, Baltimore.

Huckstep, R. L. (1971) Neglected traumatic dislocation of the hip. *J. Bone Joint Surg.*, (Br), **53–B**, 355–61.

Index